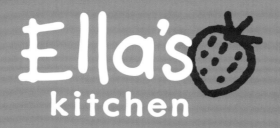

Ella's kitchen

the First Foods Book

For the 130 million babies born this year. Eat well, grow strong – for this world is yours.

Paul + Alison Lindley

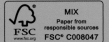
MIX
Paper from
responsible sources
FSC® C008047

First published in Great Britain
in 2015 by Hamlyn, an imprint of
Octopus Publishing Group Ltd,
Carmelite House
50 Victoria Embankment
London, EC4Y 0DZ
www.octopusbooks.co.uk

An Hachette UK Company
www.hachette.co.uk

ISBN 9780600629252

A CIP catalogue record for this book is
available from the British Library

Typeset in Cooper Light and Ella's Kitchen®
Printed and bound in China

Created by Ella's Kitchen and Harris + Wilson

27 26 25 24 23 22 21 20 19 18

Recipe development: Nicola Graimes
Art direction, design + styling: Anita Mangan
Design assistant: Ella McLean
Photographer: Jonathan Cherry
Illustrations: Parker Williams Design
Managing editor: Judy Barratt
Assistant production manager: Lucy Carter
Home economist + food stylist: Lincoln Jefferson
Photoshoot direction: Sarah Ford, Caroline Harris +
Manisha Patel

Disclaimer Children under the age of 6 months with
a family history of nut allergy, asthma, eczema or any
other type of allergy are advised to avoid eating dishes that
contain nuts. Check with a healthcare professional to make
sure you know which ingredients to avoid if you have a
child with allergies. Check all packaging for allergy advice
and use clean surfaces and utensils to avoid allergens
sneaking into your cooking. Never give whole nuts to
children under the age of 5 years in case of choking.
Some recipes contain honey. It is advised not to feed
honey to children under 12 months old. Every care should
be taken when cooking with and for children. Neither the
author nor the publisher can accept any liability for any
consequences arising from the use of this book, or the
information contained herein.

Publisher's notes
Standard level spoon measures are used in the recipes:

1 tablespoon = one 15 ml spoon
1 teaspoon = one 5 ml spoon
1 ice cube = one 15 ml spoon

Both metric and imperial measurements are given
for the recipes. Use one set of measurements only,
not a mixture of both.

Ovens should be preheated to the specified temperature.
For a fan-assisted oven, follow the manufacturer's
instructions to adjust the cooking time and temperature.

Medium-sized ingredients and pans and medium-strength
cheese have been used throughout unless otherwise
specified. Herbs are fresh unless otherwise specified.
Use low-salt stock, and avoid adding salt to recipes.

Freezing and storage
Freeze food in a freezer set at -18°C (0°F).
See pages 17 + 19 for further storage
and freezing information.

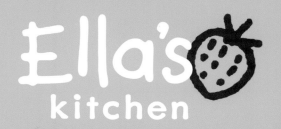

Ella's kitchen

the First Foods Book

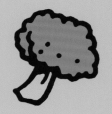

130 yummy recipes
from weaning to the big table

hamlyn

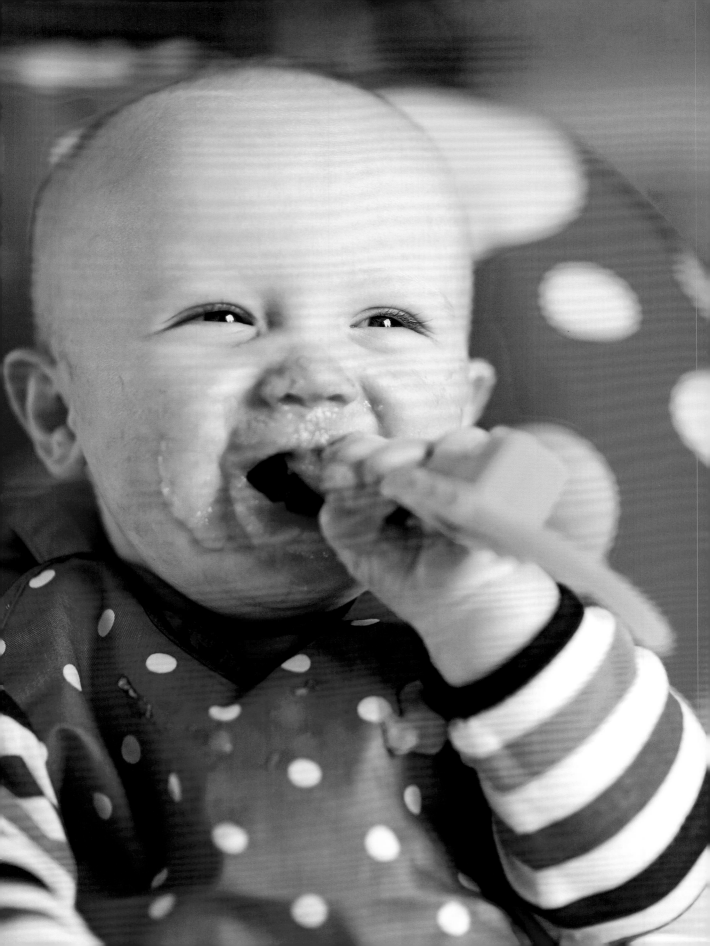

Contents

Foreword by Ella's dad

I look across the dinner table and see Ella, now 15 years old, talking about her day and I wonder where the years have gone. Fifteen years ago a high chair sat in that exact same spot, while a noisy toddler played loudly with her food; earlier still, it was the place of the first moments of her weaning journey.

Like any teenage girl, Ella can be selective about her culinary likes and dislikes, but she is always willing to try new things. Sometimes she discovers new tastes she loves (and sometimes she doesn't!). I like to think her willingness is the result of the ways in which we encouraged her to try new tastes and textures during the earliest moments, when *every* mouthful was an adventure.

Weaning can be one of the most enjoyable, but also the most frustrating and stressful times for both grown-ups and children. In the end only your instinct knows what works for you and your baby. The most important thing we've learned is that weaning is easiest when it's fun and messy and silly; when eating becomes an extension of play. I also believe that children are more likely to develop a lifelong love of food if they can build a relationship that puts food squarely into a social context – associating it with interactivity, eye contact, fun, enjoyment and being surrounded by the people they love.

Ella's weaning experience led directly to the seed of the idea that became Ella's Kitchen – that of aiming to provide healthy, handy and fun foods for children. This book joins you at the very beginning of your baby's foody journey. It puts you in charge, gives you choices, and through its tips and advice aims to help you develop the confidence to follow your instinct.

The whole Ella's Kitchen team has been involved in creating *The Purple One* – offering tips, advice and recipes. We hope you enjoy every second of using it as much as we have enjoyed creating it.

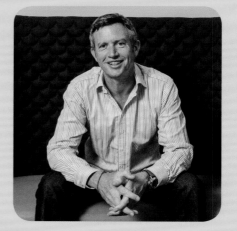

Keep smiling

Paul

Paul, Ella's dad

Follow me on Twitter: @Paul_Lindley

Foreword by Ella's mum

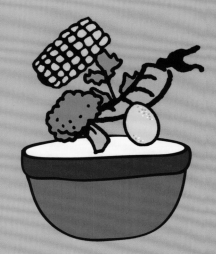

When you think about it, we actually have very little say in when our babies decide to reach many of the early milestones in their lives – from the first smile to sitting up on their own, babies tend to lead the way. Although we can't directly influence a baby's growing appetite, and babies will give their own signals about when they're ready to wean, the precise day of first weaning, and what your baby eats, is down to you.

I remember well the big countdown to Ella's first 'solids' – some baby rice. Then, Paul and I set out our weekly plan for introducing all the various puréed fruits and vegetables. We were lucky – Ella enjoyed so many of her first foods. Her favourites were carrot, parsnip and banana; and I remember very distinctly how she turned up her nose at tomatoes and avocado – both of which she now loves! Her early words were foody-based – 'more!' came first, then 'pick' for milk and 'boshstich' for breakfast.

We tried to make the whole mealtime experience as fun as possible with lots of silly songs, spoon 'choo-choo' trains, and smiles. When her baby brother, Paddy, came along, Ella fed him his first mouthful. She loved feeling involved. Paddy loved banana just as his sister had done, as well as most vegetables, and hot porridge! I clearly remember that mealtimes with him were a lot messier!

If I had one piece of advice for new mums, it would be to keep talking – to each other, to friends and to family. Paul and I had plenty of anxieties when we weaned our two – were they eating enough? Why did they love one thing one week and scowl at it the next? Were they getting enough of the right foods? Weaning is such an emotive issue – share your worries and concerns, and your ideas and recipes, too. You're part of a wonderful community of knowledge and understanding. Whatever your weaning experiences, if you keep talking you'll soon learn that every baby is different and that no matter what anxieties you're facing this day, this week or this month, you're certainly not alone.

Good luck and – most of all – have fun!

Alison
x
Alison, Ella's mum

Our first foods book

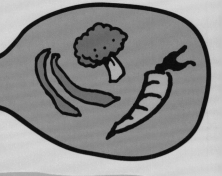

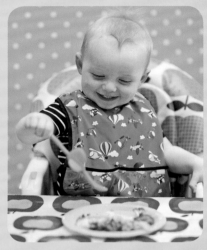

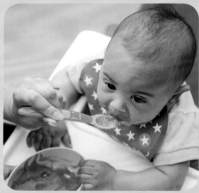

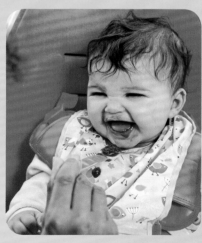

A bit about this book

You and your baby are about to embark on an amazing exploration of taste and texture, and we want to support you every step of the way. At Ella's Kitchen, our aim is to take the stress out of weaning so that you can create confident, happy mealtimes. We like to think of weaning as a journey of discovery for you and your baby – a sensory adventure that is packed with colour, and full of delicious, messy and noisy experiences.

Every baby is different and our book is all about helping you decide what's best for you and your family. We've given you lots of information and advice so that you can make informed choices about when and how to wean your baby, including how to read his or her own weaning signs. We've worked hard to develop recipes that will delight all your baby's senses and we hope that the extra tips, activities and games will make your baby's weaning journey a taste-tingling experience that starts with the very first mouthful.

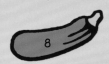

Meet the experts

We've worked closely with a number of experts to make sure our recipes are as good for your baby as possible. Here are our recipe superstars:

Claire Baseley is an Infant Nutritionist. She's helped us make sure all our ingredients are really good for tiny tummies and growing bodies.

Nicola Graimes is an award-winning cookery author, specializing in children's nutrition. She's helped us write all the book's delicious recipes.

Dr Carmel Houston-Price is a Developmental Psychologist who works with us to understand the role of the five senses in the way a baby develops healthy attitudes towards food.

Sally Luckraft is our Food Developer. She makes all Ella's yummy new stuff. She's helped make sure our recipes will tingle little taste buds.

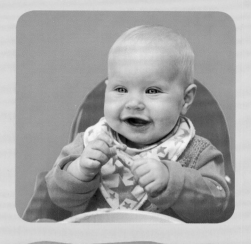

Top tips from our friends

We asked lots of Ella's Friends for their best weaning advice. Here are their top four nuggets of wisdom:

Go at your own pace It's so easy to compare your baby to all the others you know, but every baby is different and will be ready for new experiences at different times. Let *your* little one set the pace.

Love the mess Messy little faces and sticky little hands are inevitable – and they are the best signs of a fun mealtime.

The more the merrier Parents, grandparents and siblings – let everyone take a turn helping during this exciting time in your baby's life; your baby will love it!

Be kind to your time Plan your meals, shop online or locally, and learn recipe cheats (look out for our shortcuts) – that way you'll have extra time to really enjoy the weaning experience with your baby.

Key to icons

At the top of every recipe, you'll find a combination of the following symbols to help make the job of weaning your baby as easy as it can be.

makes **30** spoons — How many teaspoons the recipe makes

makes **16** ice cubes — How many ice cubes the recipe makes

makes **6** — How many pieces the recipe makes

serves **4** — How many little ones the recipe serves

serves **2+2** adults + kids — How many adults and little ones this family recipe serves

prep **10** minutes — How long the ingredients take to prepare

cook **10** minutes — How long the recipe takes to cook

How to start your baby's weaning journey

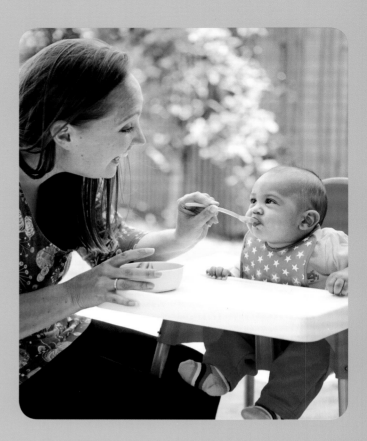

What is weaning?

Weaning is the exciting time when babies stop being wholly reliant on breastmilk or formula and begin their foody adventures.

Knowing when to begin

Advice about when to begin weaning varies all over the world. Some countries, such as the UK and USA, advise introducing solids at around 6 months old, when a baby's digestive system is usually developed enough to cope with foods other than milk. Other countries, however, suggest beginning as early as 17 weeks (4 months) old.

Everyone agrees that before 17 weeks is too young. Not only is your baby's tummy not ready then, his or her kidneys aren't yet strong enough to cope with an increased workload.

Every baby is unique, so it's impossible to be prescriptive about *the* right time for babies in general. That's why it's really important you look for the signs your own baby gives you that he or she might be gearing up for some solids – we've put those signs in the yellow box, opposite, as a handy reference.

Then, if your baby *is* ready, but is younger than 6 months old, there are certain foods you should avoid giving, as they may cause allergies or make your baby poorly. We've listed these for you on page 23.

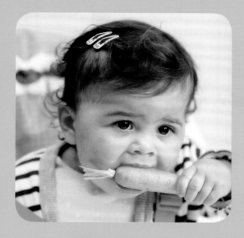

It's all about taste

At 6 months old weaning is more about taste than it is about nutrition – your baby is still getting essential nutrients from breastmilk or formula. With taste in mind, the more variety babies try in the first few weeks of weaning, the more likely they are to become good little eaters later on.

Of course, your baby might not like every new taste you present. Don't give up! You may need to offer a new taste on up to 10 separate occasions – or more – before your little one learns to love what you're giving. Keep trying, but don't force the issue. Try to make weaning a relaxed and happy time.

Some parents worry their baby isn't getting enough food in the early weeks of weaning. Try to relax. Your baby's tummy really is still tiny and milk continues to be *the* primary source of nutrition for a good while yet. As long as your baby is drinking milk, and you and your health visitor are happy your baby is growing well, you're doing fine.

Your baby's weaning signs

There are some common myths about when babies are ready to wean. For example, chewing fists, reaching for other people's food, waking in the night and wanting more milk can just be signals that your baby is doing all the normal things that babies do. They may not mean that your baby is ready for solid food at all. Babies are probably ready to start weaning when they can:

☺ Hold their head straight up on their own, and sit confidently with support.

☺ Show good hand–eye coordination, getting all their favourite toys – among other things – into their mouths.

Trust your instinct and you'll know when the time is right. Then, if when you start your baby just pushes out what you give, don't worry – wait a week or two and try again.

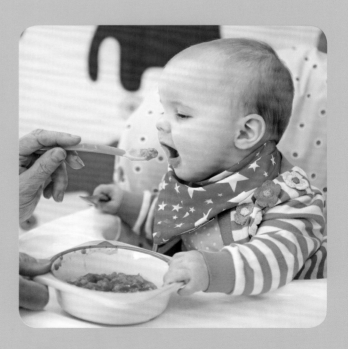

Foods to avoid

When you begin the weaning journey, not every food is good for your baby's tiny tummy. As well as the common allergens (see p.23), the following are foods you need to be extra-specially careful about.

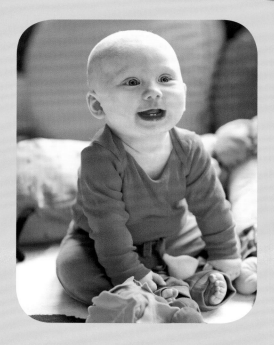

Added salt Little ones under a year old need less than 1 g of salt – or 0.4 g of sodium – a day, so added salt is a no-no. Look out! Processed foods not intended for babies, such as pasta sauces and breakfast cereals, could have lots of added salt in them; and stock cubes, too.

Added sugar Your baby is sweet enough, so avoid adding sugar in your cooking. Natural sugars in fruits provide plenty of sweetness – any more could lead to tooth decay or an unhealthy sweet tooth.

Honey Bears may like honey, but little ones shouldn't try it until they reach 1 year old, as it contains bacteria that could be harmful to tiny tummies.

Whole nuts Whole nuts, including peanuts, are easy to choke on. Don't give them until your child is over 5 years old.

Low-fat foods Low-fat yogurt, fromage frais, cheese or spreads are not 'baby's choice'. Babies need fat – it's a *reeeally* important source of calories and vitamins. You may be able to introduce low-fat foods after your little one's second birthday, but check with your doctor first.

Some fish + shellfish Some fish, including shark, marlin and swordfish, can contain high levels of mercury. Avoid giving these for the first year and after that only in small amounts. Shellfish can carry a risk of food poisoning if it's undercooked, so be very, very careful to cook it properly all the way through!

Eggs Until your baby is 1 year old, give well-cooked eggs only – there is a tiny chance of salmonella in runny eggs.

Unpasteurized + blue cheeses Soft, unpasteurized cheeses, such as Brie and Camembert, and 'mouldy' or 'blue' cheeses, such as Stilton, carry a small risk of food poisoning and are best saved for after your baby's all-important first birthday.

Your baby's milk

Up until the age of 6 months, little ones get all the nutrients they need from breastmilk or formula milk. After 6 months, solid food starts to play a more important role in growth and development and your baby's daily milk intake will start to plateau. Between 6 months and a year, babies still need around 500–600 ml (17 fl oz–1 pint) of breastmilk or formula each day.

You can use cow's milk in cooking once your baby reaches 6 months old, but don't introduce cow's milk as a drink until after a year (see p.23), and then only if it is full fat. You may be able to introduce semi-skimmed milk from 2 years old.

Nutritionist know-how

'If, at 6 months old, your baby goes off milk when you start on food, don't panic! Use the baby's usual milk in your cooking, too – add it to rice pudding, macaroni cheese or custard to pack in those essential nutrients.'

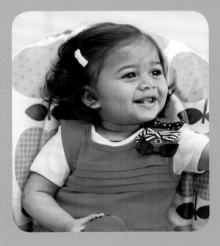

Introducing other drinks

At the start of weaning, breastfed babies can reach their fluid requirements from milk alone (formula-fed babies may need a top-up of cooled, once-boiled water in hot weather). From 6 months, *as well as* your baby's usual milk, you can introduce water from a mains tap, in a baby cup or beaker. (Never use mineral water, as it can have high salt levels.) You can also give unconcentrated, pure fruit juice diluted 1 part juice to 10 parts water (brush tiny teeth regularly, though) at mealtimes. Always avoid squash and cordial, as they contain high amounts of processed sugar.

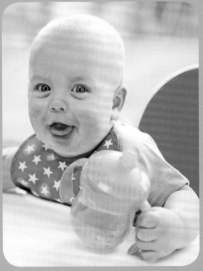

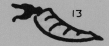

Good little eaters

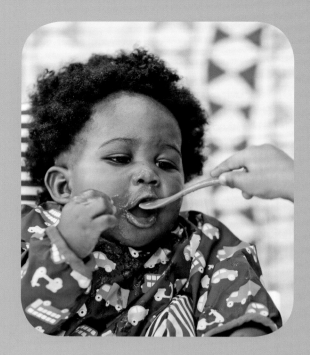

We want your little one to develop a lifelong positive relationship with food. Here are a few ways to set your baby off on the right track.

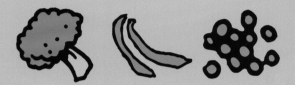

Starting with savoury

Starting weaning with green and white veg can help little ones get used to more bitter flavours early on. We've given you step-by-step guidance on one way to approach a savoury first 2 weeks on pages 24–5.

Variety, variety, variety

Offering a variety of appropriate foods and textures is super-important. A rainbow of colours (see right), different sources of proteins, carbohydrates and fats, and different herbs and spices will encourage your baby to accept new foods as he or she grows up, even into adulthood. Try to offer your baby different tastes every day.

Baby knows best

Most babies know when they've had enough to eat. Follow your baby's lead. To tell you that enough is enough, babies might turn away their head, spit out their food, or push away the bowl or spoon.

Taking a turn

As soon as possible, put a spoon in your baby's little hand to have a go – it's a great way to learn the ropes!

Happy about food

Here are some more ideas on ways to make your baby's mealtimes fun:

☺ **It's a rainbow** Presenting lots of colourful foods makes dishes look more appealing – and lots of colours indicate all-round nutritional content.

☺ **Story time** Make up stories and songs involving broccoli trees, cauliflower sheep, strawberry hedgehogs…

☺ **Pick me up** Give whole or chopped-up veg and fruit to your little one to hold – little fingers love to explore the textures. And encourage messy play with food, which can help babies develop a positive foody relationship.

☺ **Family experiences** Eat together whenever you can, showing that mealtimes are sociable occasions.

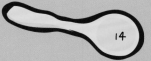

Good in every sense

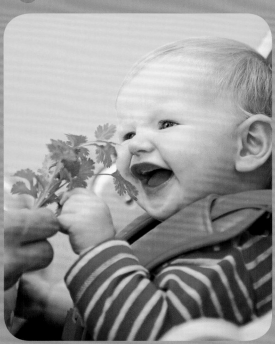

Our research has shown us that little ones who are able to experience veggies and fruit using all their senses are much more likely to eat those foods when mealtimes come around and to have a lifelong positive relationship with food. That's why we've put lots of ideas throughout the book for sensorial games you can try together. Let's play!

Feed the senses

Tongue-ticklingly tasty...

Babies have three times more taste buds than grown-ups, so trying new foods is really exciting for them. Our recipes use lots of herbs and spices and exciting ingredients to get tongues zinging!

Smells super...

Our sense of smell is essential to our sense of taste. Encourage your baby to smell food before eating it to get the full flavour experience. Mmmmm...

Touchy feely...

As little ones grow up, they recognize different foods by texture. Being able to hold ingredients and finger foods is important for this developmental step.

Looks lovely...

When discovering food, colour and shape are really important – offer a rainbow of foods in different shapes and sizes.

Sounds scrummy...

Foods make all sorts of sounds: carrots snap, onions sizzle, sauces bubble... Listen to the sounds of cooking and eating together, and make lots of 'yumminess' sounds during mealtimes. (Download some 'Tasty Tunes' from our website, too!)

Store-cupboard superheroes

Juggling a baby and everyday life is hard work! Even the most organized wonder-mums and super-dads can get caught short.

We believe that with a few store-cupboard essentials tucked away in the kitchen, anyone can whip up a delicious, nutritious meal for a little one in no time at all.

Pasta, rice + couscous

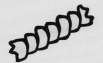

These are perfect accompaniments, but also delicious stirred through a sauce (see below).

Canned tomatoes + tomato purée

Add a few herbs and there's your sauce!

Canned pulses

Butter beans and lentils provide texture and flavour, and are fantastic sources of protein.

Canned fish

Sardines and salmon can provide instant sources of protein and healthy fats.

Rolled oats

These are brilliant for simple breakfasts, or mixed with fruit for a pudding.

Dried herbs + spices

Cinnamon, oregano, thyme and turmeric can transform simple dishes.

Dried fruit

Raisins, sultanas and dark, unsulphured apricots make perfect toddler finger foods; or whiz them with some yogurt for an instant pudding.

Eggs

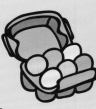

A mashed-up boiled egg or well-cooked scramble provides instant nutrition. Mixed with flour and some milk, eggs make a batter for pancakes, too.

Frozen veg

Veggies that are always fresh! A bag of frozen peas or broccoli means that supergreen nutrition is always at hand.

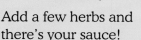
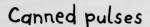
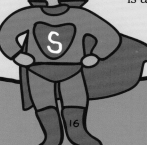

Safe + secure

Following a few simple rules helps keep little ones as safe as possible on their weaning adventure.

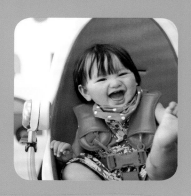

Wipe clean

Keep surfaces, chopping boards and utensils spotlessly clean. Use separate chopping boards for meat and veg.

Clean hands

Always wash your own hands before preparing any food. Then, check that your baby's hands are clean before eating. It's never too early to get babies into the habit of hand-washing before a meal.

Wash, peel + scrape

Wash all ingredients and either peel or scrub away tough skins before you cook.

Clean bowls + spoons

If your baby is younger than 6 months, sterilize all your feeding equipment (see p.18). After that, just make sure everything is washed really well in hot, soapy water and rinsed in clean water.

Hot, hot, hot

Cook or reheat food so it's piping hot all the way through, then stir it and cool it to a lukewarm temperature. Test it against your bottom lip to make sure it's just right for your baby. Never reheat cooked food more than once, and never refreeze food that's been frozen and then defrosted.

Two's company

Never leave your baby alone when eating or drinking – you need to be around in case of any mishaps, including choking.

Be cool

If you want to refrigerate (or freeze) food, make sure it's completely cold first. Cool it quickly – within 2 hours of cooking – by standing the container of food in a bowl of cold water. Once it's thoroughly cold, pop it in the fridge (or freezer).

Store safely

Keep cooked and raw meats covered and away from each other. Place cooked foods above raw foods in the fridge, and put non-meat foods on a separate fridge shelf.

Keep it fresh

Here are some guidelines for storing freshly made foods:

 In the fridge: 2 days in an airtight container

 In the freezer: up to 1 month at -18°C/0°F

 Cakes + bakes: in the cupboard for up to 3–4 days in an airtight container

Your weaning kitchen

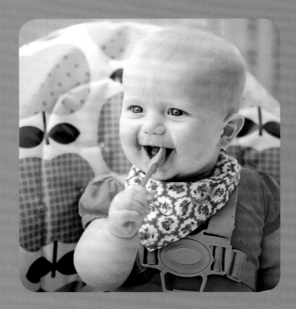

What you'll need

So, before you get started, here's our guide to a few essentials you'll need in your kitchen to make it easier to prepare and store your baby's food.

- ☺ **Vegetable peeler** because you'll be doing a *lot* of peeling

- ☺ **Sharp paring knife** to chop things up nice and small

- ☺ **Small saucepans** that are perfect sizes for reheating little portions

- ☺ **Steamer**… but that needs a section all of its own (see opposite)

- ☺ **Sieve** to strain fruit, catch naughty pips and help get rid of tough skins

- ☺ **Hand blender** or **food processor** to whiz your baby's food to the right texture (food processors are better for tougher skins on veggies)

- ☺ **Potato masher** for when your little one moves on from purée

- ☺ **Sterilizer** for spoons and bowls, but only if you're weaning before your baby is 6 months old (you can sterilize in boiling water if you prefer)

- ☺ **Ice-cube trays** for storing purées in the freezer in portions

- ☺ **Freezer bags** for storing frozen purée cubes, or for freezing finger foods

- ☺ **Labels + marker pen** so you know what's what and when you made it

- ☺ **Beakers + cups** to help your baby move on from a bottle

- ☺ **Plastic spoons + bowls** for feeding time itself

- ☺ **High chair** or **booster seat** so your little one can sit at the table

- ☺ **Bibs** – we like the plastic ones with a tray to catch the bits

- ☺ **Face cloths** or **muslins** for wiping messy hands and faces

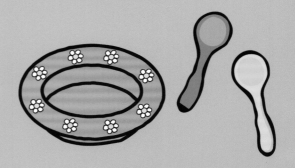

Getting steamy!

Steaming food is the best way to preserve nutrients and keep flavour locked in. Steam veggies until just tender – they're less tasty when they're mushy. Here are some steaming methods to choose from.

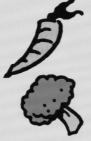

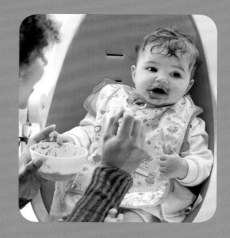

Dedicated steamer Some steamers are fancy electrical tiered units, while others look like a stack of saucepans with holes in.

Steamer basket These are holey baskets with little feet – they look like little spaceships. You put them in a saucepan with a little boiling water, cover and steam away.

Colander Pop your colander in a pan with a little water and cover it with a lid – hey presto, the steamer you never knew you had!

Microwave Put a little water in a microwave bowl, add the veggies and cover with clingfilm. Pierce the film and then zap in the microwave until the veggies are tender (about 2–3 minutes for leafy greens and 5–6 minutes for chopped root veg – but check your user guide).

Our friends say...

'Once my baby had moved on from single purées, I loved mixing and matching my ice cubes (see below) into interesting flavour combinations!'

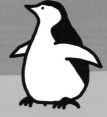

Freezer essentials

Freezing your baby's food in batches can help make weaning *soooo* much easier, especially in the early stages. The quantities of our purée recipes for 6 and 7 months are given in ice cubes (1 ice cube = about 3 teaspoons). A guide to portion size is given at the start of each chapter to help you decide how much to defrost.

☺ Make sure your purées are completely cooled (see p.17) before you put them in the freezer.

☺ Label freezer bags with the name of the food and the date you made it.

☺ Use frozen food within 1 month.

☺ Defrost your food completely before reheating it. The safest ways to defrost are covered in the fridge overnight, or in a microwave.

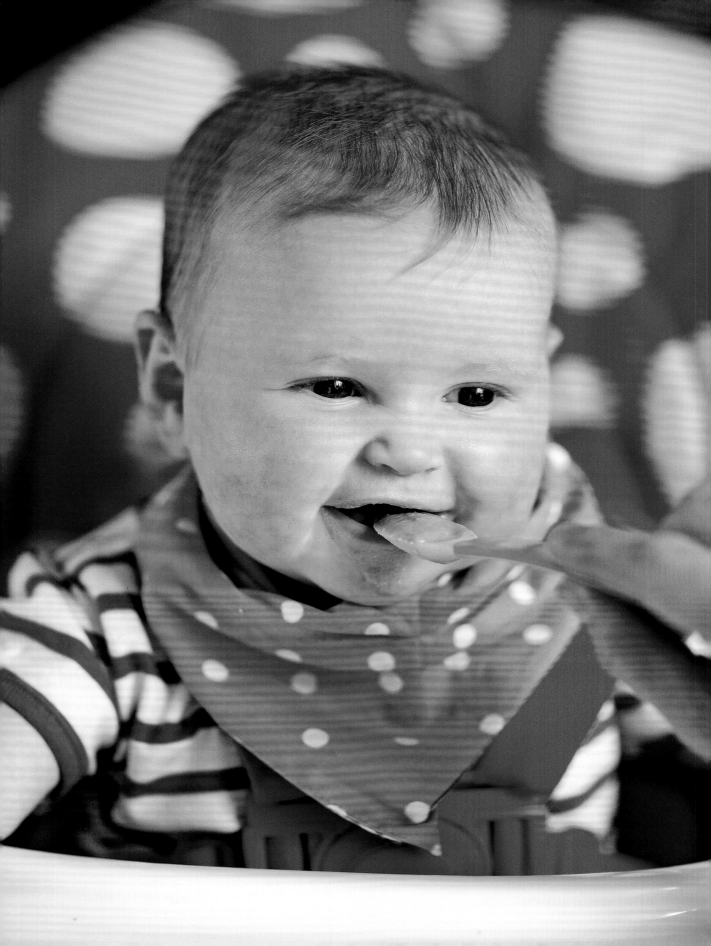

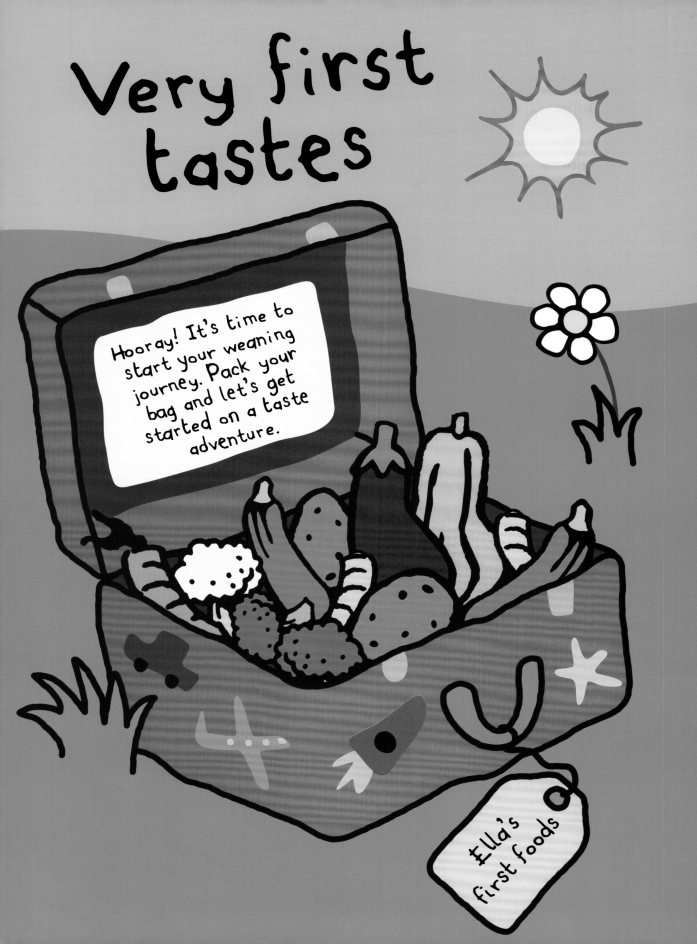

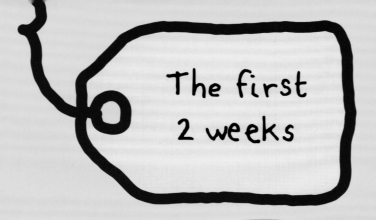

The first 2 weeks

Your baby is ready and it's time to get started. Here is the essential information you need to make sure you both put your best weaning feet forward.

Best first foods

Research tells us that offering only veggies for the first 2 weeks of weaning is the very best way to entice tiny taste buds to love a whole range of flavours. The table on the following page is our step-by-step guide to this 'veg first' approach. Don't be surprised if your baby screws up that little face at first – breastmilk is sweet, so savoury flavours may be a bit of a surprise. Go gently, and don't worry if your baby seems to eat very little – remember, it's all about taste for now.

If your baby isn't 6 months old yet, there are some foods that you need to avoid because they increase the risk of little ones developing allergies. Take a look at our box (opposite) for a handy guide, and consult your doctor if you're unsure.

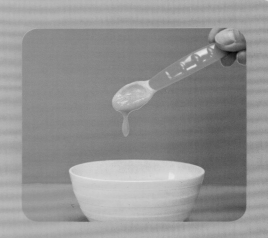

Tips on texture

Although they can't chew yet, babies can move food from the front to the back of their mouths, and swallow.

We often call very first foods 'solids', but there's really very little that's solid about them just yet! Try to create the texture of double cream or runny honey (like in the picture, above) in a perfectly smooth purée. You'll probably need to loosen the consistency of the puréed food with a little boiled water, or with a little of your baby's usual milk, if you prefer.

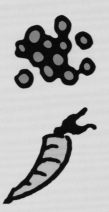

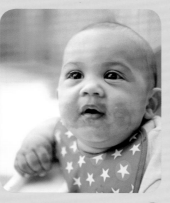

Perfect timing

A new flavour once a day is just right for the first 2 weeks. Pick a time to start when your baby isn't too hungry – usually just after or during a milk feed – and not too tired. Leave plenty of time to enjoy the experience – don't start weaning when you've planned a busy day.

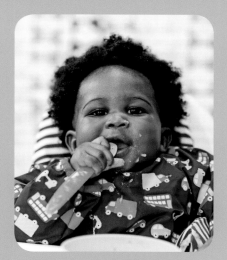

How much?

At the start of weaning, babies still get their nutrition from their usual milk – around 500–600 ml (17 fl oz–1 pint) a day – so try not to worry about how much solid food goes in. Right now, it's all about the flavour variety (and getting used to a spoon). Defrost just 1 ice cube at a time (see p.19 for how to do this safely), because a weaning spoonful or two is often plenty at the start. Take your baby's lead (see p.14).

Allergy essentials

Before 6 months of age, babies' digestive systems are very sensitive to the effects of certain 'allergen' foods. Even after 6 months, if you have a family history of allergies such as eczema or asthma, or of any food allergy, check with your doctor before you offer any of the following.

Allergen foods to avoid

☹ Cereals containing gluten

☹ Eggs

☹ Fish + shellfish

☹ Nuts (including peanuts)

☹ Soybeans

☹ Celery + celeriac

☹ Cow's milk + other dairy products

☹ Mustard

☹ Sesame

Signs of an allergic reaction

Always keep an eye out for potential allergic reactions. Signs to watch for are:

☹ Irritated skin or a red rash, especially on your baby's face

☹ Swollen lips + mouth

☹ Runny nose + watery eyes

☹ Tummy upsets, including pain, vomiting or very runny poo

☹ Difficulty breathing (extreme cases)

If you're at all worried, consult your doctor or health visitor; and if your baby shows any signs of breathing difficulties, go straight to hospital.

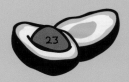

Our first tastes weaning planner

We know those very first steps on your baby's weaning journey can feel a bit daunting. To help you, we've created this 2-week weaning planner. It uses a 'veg first' weaning approach (see p.14) to help get your baby used to savoury rather than sweet tastes as early as possible. Stay focused on building your little one's positive relationship with food – follow your instinct, listen to your baby, and most of all have *lots* of messy fun.

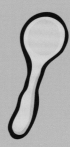

1–2 spoonfuls just after lunchtime milk*

	Day 1	Day 2	Day 3	Day 4	Day 5	Day 6	Day 7
Week 1	potatoes	broccoli	cauliflower	green beans	cabbages	avocado	peas
Week 2	courgettes	Brussels sprouts	aubergine	carrots	parsnips	butternut squash	swede

* or, whatever time suits you and your baby best!

Using the planner

The planner suggests *one new veggie taste once a day, every day,* for the first 2 weeks. All the recipes for these purées are on pages 26–9.

We think just after a lunchtime milk feed is a good time to start your baby's very first tastes – but work with what suits you and your baby best. And remember that tiny amounts – just one or two weaning spoonfuls at a time – are probably enough.

Keep up the milk

As the first steps in weaning are just about taste, it's really important that babies keep to their usual routine and amounts (see p.23) when it comes to milk feeds – they still need all the goodness in breastmilk or formula to keep them healthy.

You can substitute your baby's usual milk for the water in the recipe when you need to thin a purée, if you prefer.

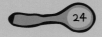

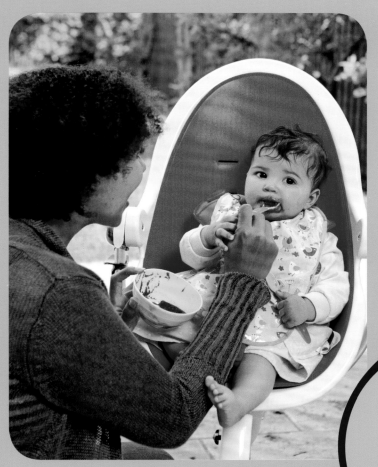

After the first 2 weeks

Keep offering veg or fruit (see below) one at a time and, when you feel ready, move on to simple combinations. Once babies are over 6 months of age and ready for more exciting combos, they can try all the yummy recipes in the following chapter.

Our friends say...

'I wanted my baby to associate her high chair with having lots of fun, so in the week before we started weaning, I'd sit her in it to play games and sing songs. Then, when the food came, she knew that was going to be fun, too!'

Other favourite very first foods

We think variety is so important for your baby. Below are some other favourite first tastes he or she might like. All of these fruits and veggies need to be peeled, and all but banana will need to be cooked until tender so that you can whiz the flesh into a super-soft purée (adding a little of your baby's usual milk if you need to). For banana, mash until smooth with the back of a fork and mix it with a little breastmilk or formula so that it's not too sticky.

cucumber   sweet potatoes   pumpkin   apples   bananas   mangoes   pears   peaches   plums

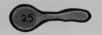

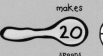

Potatoes

makes **20** spoons   cook **20** minutes

1 **potato** (about 200 g/7½ oz), such as Maris Piper, peeled and cut into 1 cm/½ inch cubes

Cook the potato in a small saucepan of boiling water for 20 minutes until very tender, then drain, reserving the cooking water. Transfer the potato to a bowl and gradually add 60 ml/ 2½ fl oz of the reserved cooking water, mashing with a fork between each addition until the purée is loose enough that a little on the end of a spoon falls off sideways without any shaking.

Broccoli

makes **20** spoons   cook **10** minutes

½ small head **broccoli** (about 130 g/ 4½ oz), cut into small florets

Steam or boil the broccoli in a saucepan over a medium heat for 8 minutes until very tender. Adding 2–3 tablespoons boiled water, purée the broccoli in a food processor, or using a hand blender, until smooth.

You can thin all the purées using your baby's usual milk, if you prefer!

Cauliflower

makes **30** spoons   cook **10** minutes

⅓ small head **cauliflower** (about 140 g/5 oz), cut into small florets

Steam or boil the cauliflower in a saucepan over a medium heat for 8–10 minutes until very tender. Adding 4–5 tablespoons boiled water, purée the cauliflower in a food processor, or using a hand blender, until smooth.

Green beans

makes **20** spoons   cook **10** minutes

100 g/3½ oz **green beans**, trimmed and halved

Steam or boil the beans in a saucepan over a medium heat for about 7 minutes until very tender. Gradually adding 3–4 tablespoons boiled water, purée the beans in a food processor, or using a hand blender, until smooth. Pass the purée through a sieve to remove any fibrous pieces before serving.

Cabbages

makes **15** spoons cook **5** minutes

¼ **white cabbage** (about 130 g/4½ oz), cored and finely chopped

Steam or boil the cabbage in a saucepan over a medium heat for about 5 minutes until very tender. Adding 2–3 tablespoons boiled water, purée the cabbage in a food processor, or using a hand blender, until smooth. Pass the purée through a sieve to remove any fibrous pieces before serving.

Avocado

serves **1** cook **no cook**

1 very ripe **avocado**, peeled, stoned and chopped

Baby's usual milk (optional)

Using the back of a fork, mash the avocado until completely smooth, adding a little of your baby's usual milk if necessary. Alternatively, purée using a hand blender. (Mashed avocado won't keep, so discard any leftovers.)

Peas

makes 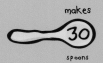 **30** spoons cook **15** minutes

150 g/5½ oz **frozen peas**

Steam or boil the peas in a saucepan over a medium heat for 10–12 minutes until completely tender. Purée the peas with 3–4 tablespoons of boiled water in a food processor, or using a hand blender, until completely smooth. Pass the purée through a sieve to remove any pieces of skin, if necessary.

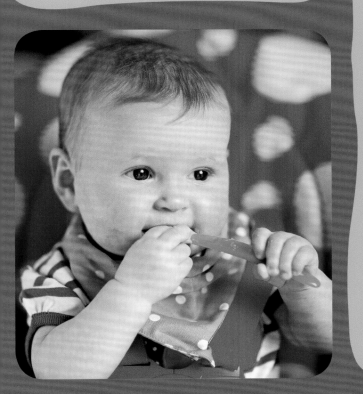

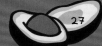

27

Courgettes

makes 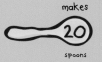 20 spoons

cook 10 minutes

1 **courgette** (about 150 g/5½ oz), halved lengthways and cut into 5 mm/¼ inch thick slices

---

Steam or boil the courgette in a saucepan over a medium heat for 8–10 minutes until completely tender. Purée in a food processor, or using a hand blender, until smooth.

Brussels sprouts

makes 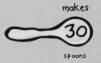 30 spoons

cook 15 minutes

150 g/5½ oz **Brussels sprouts**

Cut off the base of the sprouts and remove the outer leaves. Cut the sprouts in halves or quarters and steam over a medium heat for about 10–12 minutes until very tender (steaming is best as boiled sprouts can taste bitter). Purée the sprouts with 4–5 tablespoons of boiled water in a food processor, or using a hand blender, until smooth.

Stronger flavours add to your baby's foody adventure.

Aubergine

makes 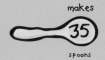 35 spoons

cook 10 minutes

1 **aubergine** (about 250 g/9 oz), cut into 1 cm/½ inch cubes

---

Steam the aubergine over a medium heat for 10 minutes until the skin and flesh are completely tender. Purée the aubergine with 2–3 tablespoons of boiled water in a food processor, or using a hand blender, until smooth. Pass the purée through a sieve to remove any pieces of skin, if necessary.

Carrots

makes 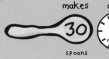 30 spoons

cook 15 minutes

3 **carrots** (about 250 g/9 oz), peeled and halved lengthways

---

Slice the carrots into half-moon shapes, 5 mm/¼ in thick. Steam or boil the carrots in a saucepan over a medium heat for 10–12 minutes until completely tender. Purée the carrots with 3–4 tablespoons of boiled water in a food processor, or using a hand blender, until completely smooth.

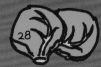

Parsnips

makes **30** spoons

cook **15** minutes

2 **parsnips** (about 350g/12 oz), peeled and cut into 1 cm/½ inch cubes

Steam or boil the parsnips in a saucepan over a medium heat for 10–12 minutes until very tender. Purée the parsnips with 150–175 ml/5–6 fl oz boiled water in a food processor, or using a hand blender, until smooth.

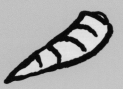

Butternut squash

makes **30** spoons

cook **15** minutes

½ **butternut squash** (about 250 g/9 oz), peeled

Cut the squash in half and scoop out the seeds. Cut the flesh into 1 cm/½ inch cubes. Steam or boil the squash in a saucepan over a medium heat for 15 minutes, or until very tender. Purée the squash with 4–5 tablespoons of boiled water in a food processor, or using a hand blender, until smooth.

Swede

makes **30** spoons

cook **20** minutes

½ **swede** (about 250 g/9 oz), peeled and cut into 1 cm/½ inch cubes

Steam or boil the swede cubes in a saucepan over a medium heat for about 20 minutes until completely tender. Purée the swede with 4–5 tablespoons of boiled water in a food processor, or using a hand blender, until smooth.

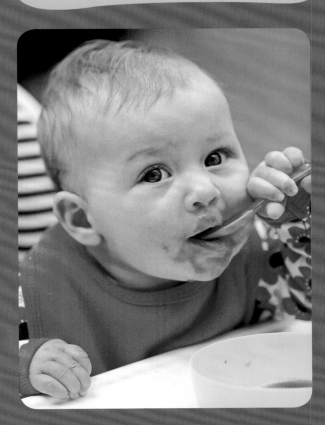

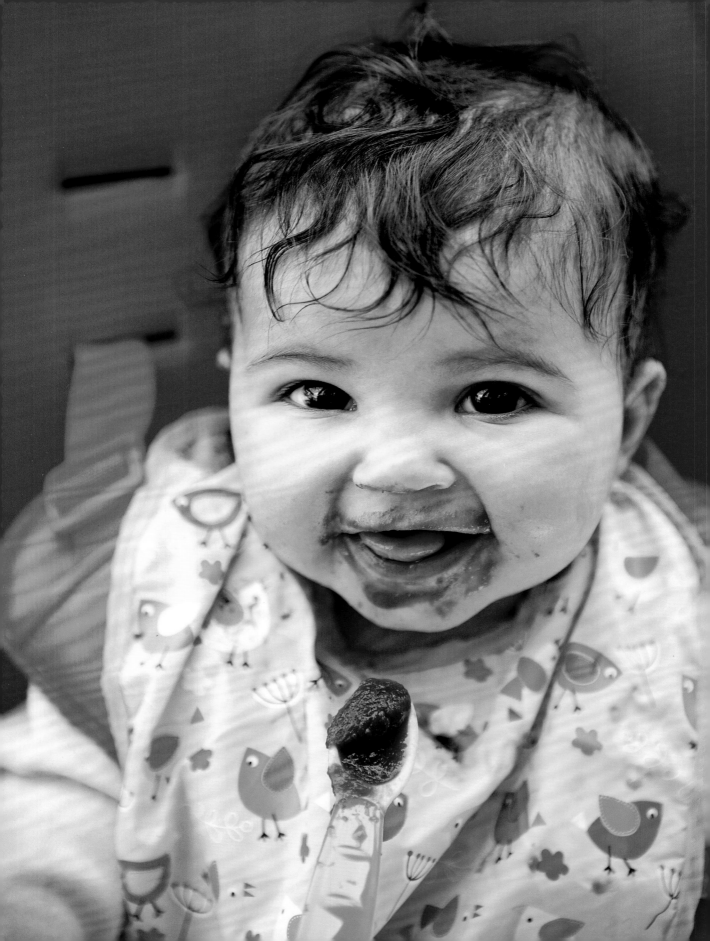

Smoothly does it

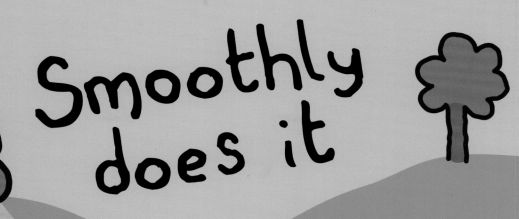

Now you're 6 months old you can try some new and exciting taste combinations! Come on, what are you waiting for?

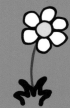

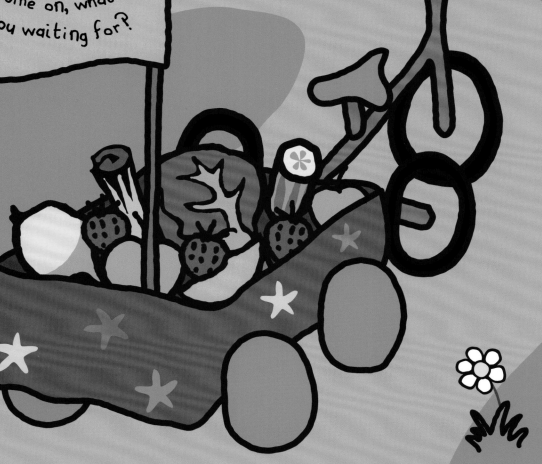

From 6 months

Now that your little one has started to learn about the world of food and how individual flavours taste, you can begin to combine different flavours and introduce new food groups. All the recipes in this chapter are not only new taste experiences for your baby, they start to work in vital nutrients, too.

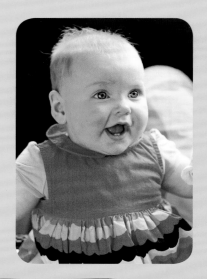

What to give

Milk is still babies' main source of nutrition and they need 500 ml (17 fl oz) of breastmilk or formula a day. Babies' natural iron stores are beginning to run a bit low around now, though, so to give an iron boost cook up dark green vegetables such as spinach, kale and broccoli; lentils are good for iron, too. Vitamin C helps babies to absorb iron, so try combining iron-rich foods with citrus fruits (see our Lentils, Squash, Oranges + Tomatoes on page 34).

At 6 months old babies are ready to discover the creamy yumminess of certain dairy foods (such as full-fat natural yogurt or fromage frais, but not milk as a drink just yet). These provide calcium for growing bones. Dairy, and pulses such as lentils, are also a good source of first protein – they are easy on tiny tummies. A pulse- or dairy-containing meal once a day gives plenty of protein to help your baby grow. Your baby can also start exploring wheat-based foods, such as pastas and cereals.

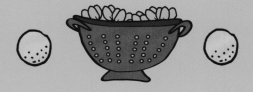

Tips on texture

At 6 months or so, babies are able to use their tongues to move food from side to side. They still need super-smooth purées with no bits and that have the consistency of double cream or runny honey (see p.22). When babies start to show signs of rolling food around their mouths in a sort of early chewing, they're ready for slightly thicker purées made using less liquid. Adding some baby rice makes the texture thicker and grainier still.

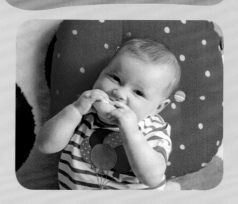

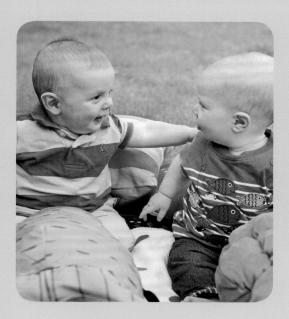

Perfect timing

Once your little one is eating well once a day, it's probably time to try 2 meals daily instead. Try lunch then tea, or breakfast then lunch – whatever works best for your family.

How much?

Even though babies grow quickly, their tummies are still teeny tiny (about the size of a baby's clenched fist). At 6 months babies might eat 1–2 ice cubes of food at each meal. Keep things relaxed and watch out for signs that your baby is ready to stop (see p.14).

Tingling taste buds

Variety is so important! Sprinkle different spices and herbs into your baby's food for taste adventures (heat dried herbs through completely, purée the leaves of any fresh herbs and don't leave woody bits). Don't forget a rainbow of veg and those different proteins from pulses and dairy, too!

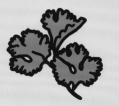

Allergy check

If you have a family history of allergies such as eczema and asthma, or of any food allergies, take care when you introduce dairy or wheat to your baby's diet (see p.23).

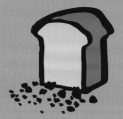

Water or milk?

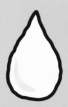

Many of the purées in this chapter suggest diluting with boiled water, but you could use cooking liquid or your baby's usual milk, if you prefer.

Lentils, squash, oranges + tomatoes

makes 14 ice cubes

prep 10 minutes

cook 20 minutes

40 g/1½ oz dried **split red lentils**, rinsed

60 g/2¼ oz **butternut squash**, peeled, deseeded and cubed

1 **tomato**, deseeded and diced

4 tablespoons **fresh orange juice**

Place the lentils and squash in a saucepan, cover with water and bring to the boil, then reduce the heat and simmer for 10 minutes, skimming off any foam. Add the tomato and cook for a further 5 minutes until everything is tender, then drain.

Purée the lentils, squash and tomato with the orange juice in a food processor, or using a hand blender, until smooth.

Leeks, cheese + potatoes

makes 18 ice cubes

prep 10 minutes

cook 25 minutes

1 tablespoon **olive oil**

1 **leek**, trimmed and chopped

1 **potato** (about 200 g/7 oz), peeled and diced

1 teaspoon **thyme leaves**

10 g/¼ oz **mature Cheddar cheese**, finely grated

Heat the oil in a saucepan over a low heat and cook the leek for 5 minutes until softened. Add the potato and thyme, cover with water, bring to the boil, then reduce the heat and simmer for 15 minutes, or until the potato is tender. Drain, reserving the cooking water. Purée the vegetables with the cheese and 6–7 tablespoons of the cooking water in a food processor, or using a hand blender, until smooth. For a smoother purée, pass it through a sieve after blending.

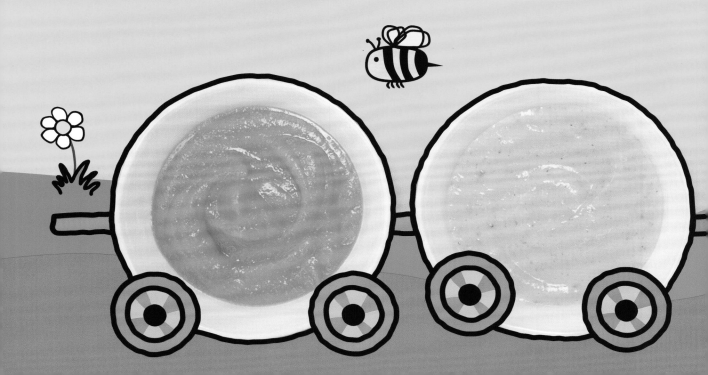

Green beans + peas

makes 8 ice cubes | **prep** 5 minutes | **cook** 10 minutes

100 g/3½ oz **green beans**, trimmed and halved

100 g/3½ oz **frozen peas**

Steam or boil the beans in a saucepan over a medium heat for 3 minutes. Add the peas and cook for a further 2–3 minutes until the vegetables are tender.

Purée the vegetables with 100 ml/ 3½ fl oz boiled water in a food processor, or using a hand blender, until the peas are completely broken down and the mixture is smooth. For a smoother purée, pass it through a sieve after blending.

Swede + parsnips

makes 13 ice cubes | **prep** 5 minutes | **cook** 20 minutes

¼ **swede** (about 100 g/3½ oz), peeled and diced

1 small **parsnip** (about 75 g/ 2½ oz), peeled and diced

5 tablespoons **baby's usual milk**

Steam or boil the swede in a saucepan over a medium heat for 15 minutes. Add the parsnip and cook for a further 5 minutes until tender. Purée with the milk in a food processor, or using a hand blender, until smooth.

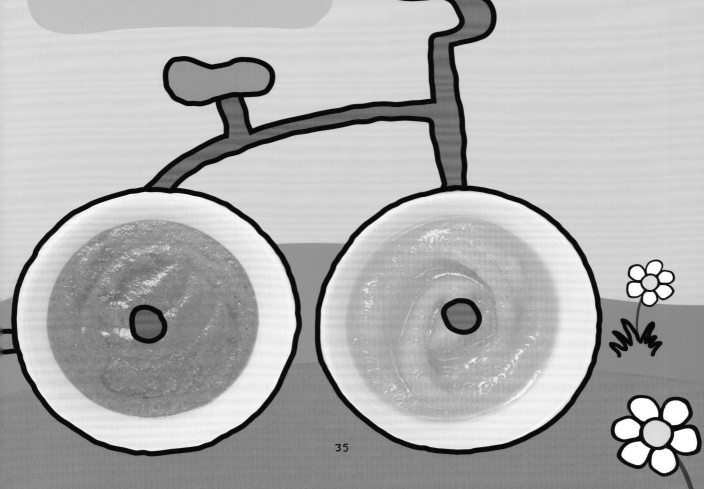

35

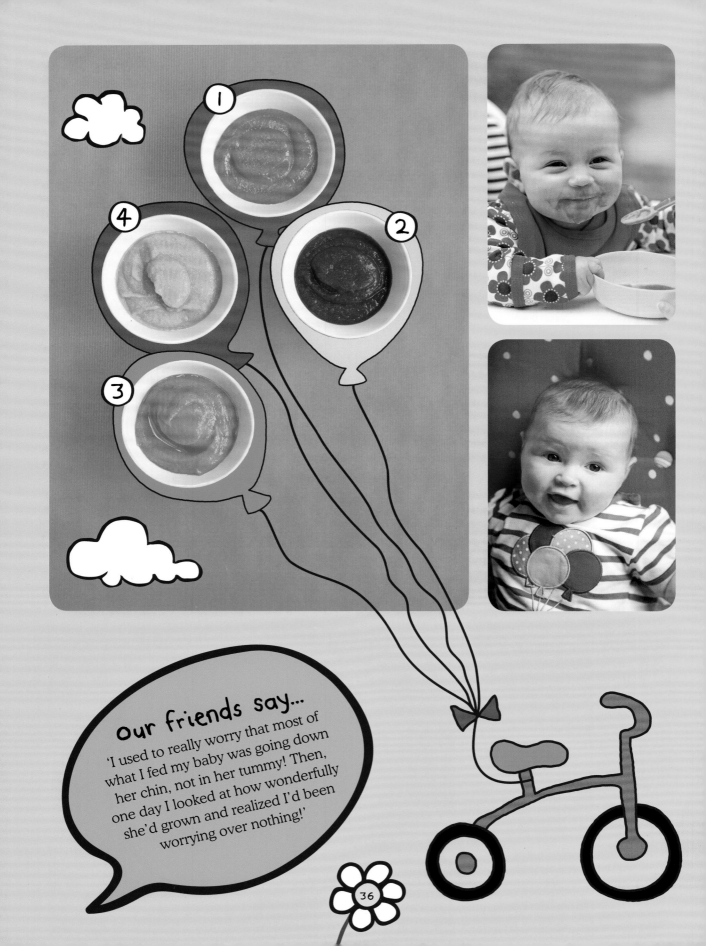

1

Sweet potatoes + red peppers

makes 17 ice cubes   **prep** 5 minutes   **cook** 15 minutes

1 **sweet potato** (about 250 g/9 oz), peeled and cubed

½ small **red pepper**, deseeded and chopped

Steam or boil the sweet potato in a saucepan over a medium heat for 5 minutes. Add the pepper and cook for 10 minutes more until the potatoes are tender and cooked through. In a food processor or using a hand blender, purée with 3–4 tablespoons boiled water until smooth.

2

Red cabbage + apples

makes 12 ice cubes   **prep** 10 minutes   **cook** 20 minutes

¼ **red cabbage** (about 70 g/2½ oz), finely chopped

2 **eating apples**, peeled, cored and cut into bite-sized pieces

Put the ingredients in a saucepan. Pour in 125 ml/4 fl oz water, cover with a lid, and bring almost to boiling point over a medium heat. Reduce the heat to low and simmer for 15–18 minutes until everything is very tender. Add a further 2–3 tablespoons boiled water, then in a food processor or using a hand blender, purée until smooth.

3

Mangoes, carrots + strawberries

makes 20 ice cubes   **prep** 10 minutes   **cook** 15 minutes

2 small **carrots** (about 120 g/4 oz), peeled and sliced

½ **mango** (about 135 g/4¾ oz), peeled, stoned and chopped

4 **strawberries**, hulled and quartered

Steam or boil the carrots in a saucepan over a medium heat for 12–15 minutes until very tender. In a food processor or using a hand blender, purée the carrots, mango and strawberries until smooth.

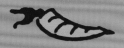

4

Butternut squash, sweetcorn + peas

  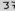

makes 21 ice cubes   **prep** 10 minutes   **cook** 15 minutes

½ **butternut squash** (about 400 g/14 oz), peeled, deseeded and cubed

60 g/2¼ oz **frozen peas**

100 g/3½ oz no-salt and no-sugar canned **sweetcorn**, drained

Steam or boil the butternut squash in a saucepan over a medium heat for 10 minutes until almost cooked. Add the peas and sweetcorn and cook for 5 minutes more until everything is tender. In a food processor or using a hand blender, purée with 5 tablespoons boiled water until smooth.

Carrots + turnips

makes **12** ice cubes | prep **5** minutes | cook **15** minutes

2 large **carrots** (about 280 g/10 oz), peeled and thinly sliced

280 g/10 oz **turnip**, peeled and diced

Steam or boil the carrots and turnip in a saucepan over a medium heat for 10–12 minutes, or until tender.

Purée the vegetables with 3 tablespoons of boiled water in a food processor, or using a hand blender, until smooth.

Peas, courgettes, mint + rice

makes **8** ice cubes | prep **5** minutes | cook **15** minutes

25 g/1 oz **white basmati rice**

1 **courgette** (about 150 g/5½ oz), diced

40 g/1½ oz **frozen peas**

4 **mint** leaves

Cook the rice according to the packet instructions until tender. Meanwhile, steam or boil the courgette over a medium heat for 5 minutes. Add the peas and cook for a further 3 minutes until the vegetables are tender. Purée the vegetables with the cooked rice, the mint and 2 tablespoons of boiled water, in a food processor, or using a hand blender, until the mixture is smooth. For a smoother purée, pass it through a sieve after blending.

Swede, carrots + cinnamon

makes **30** ice cubes | prep **5** minutes | cook **20** minutes

⅓ **swede** (about 175 g/6 oz), peeled and diced

2 **carrots** (about 150 g/5½ oz), peeled and thinly sliced

A generous pinch of **ground cinnamon**

Steam or boil the swede over a medium heat for 10 minutes. Add the carrots and cook for a further 10 minutes until the vegetables are tender. Purée with the cinnamon and 125 ml/4 fl oz boiled water in a food processor, or using a hand blender, until smooth.

Pears + avocado

serves **1** | prep **10** minutes | cook **no cook**

½ small ripe **pear**, peeled, cored and chopped

¼ small ripe **avocado**, peeled, stoned and chopped

2 tablespoons **natural yogurt** or **baby's usual milk**, plus extra if needed

A squeeze of **lemon juice**

Purée the pear, avocado, yogurt or milk and lemon juice in a food processor, or using a hand blender, until smooth, adding a little extra milk if necessary.

38

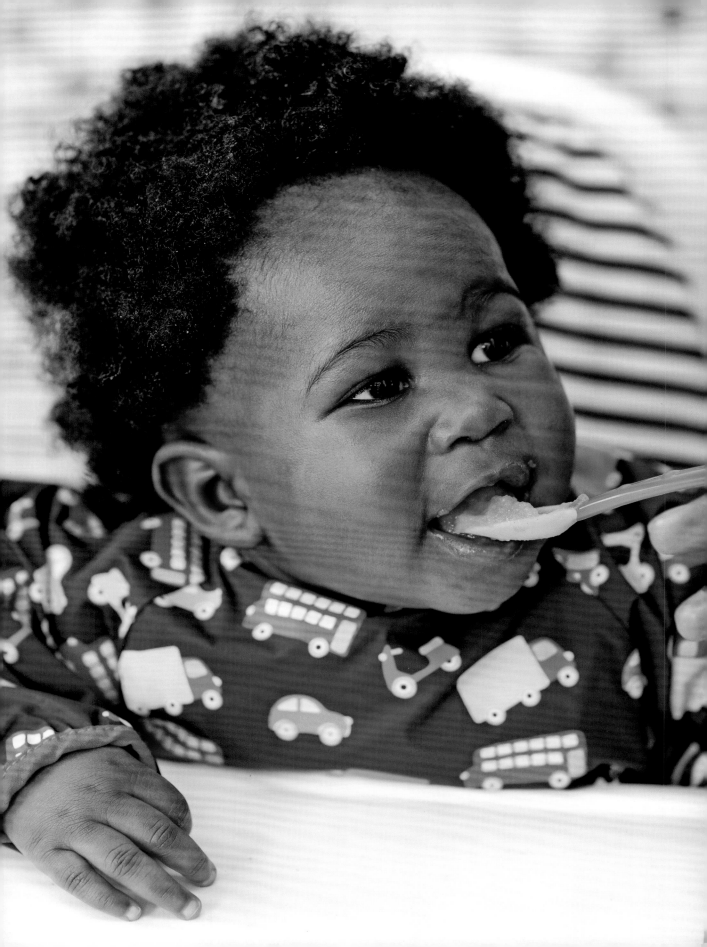

Broccoli, cauliflower + courgettes

makes 15 ice cubes | prep 10 minutes | cook 10 minutes

½ small head **broccoli** (about 150 g/5½ oz), cut into small florets

⅓ small head **cauliflower** (about 150 g/5½ oz), cut into small florets

1 **courgette** (about 150 g/5½ oz), diced

1 teaspoon chopped **parsley**

Steam or boil the vegetables in a saucepan over a medium heat for 7–8 minutes until tender. Add the parsley and heat through. Purée with 3–4 tablespoons of boiled water in a food processor, or using a hand blender, until smooth. For a smoother purée, pass it through a sieve after blending.

Oats, bananas + mixed spice

makes 12 ice cubes | prep 5 minutes | cook 10 minutes

25 g/1 oz **porridge oats**

200 ml/7 fl oz **baby's usual milk**, plus extra if needed

A large pinch of **ground mixed spice**

1 small ripe **banana**, sliced

Place the oats, milk and spice in a small saucepan and bring to the boil, then reduce to a simmer for 8–10 minutes, stirring frequently, until the oats are soft. Purée with the banana in a food processor, or using a hand blender, until smooth, adding extra milk if necessary.

Peaches + blueberries

makes 5 ice cubes | prep 5 minutes | cook no cook

3 ripe **peaches**, halved, stoned and diced

80 g/2¾ oz **blueberries**

Purée the peach and blueberries with 3 tablespoons of water in a food processor, or using a hand blender, until all the fruit skin is broken down and the mixture is smooth. To make the purée smoother, pass it through a sieve after blending.

Sweet potatoes, carrots, cheese + broccoli

makes 10 ice cubes | prep 10 minutes | cook 15 minutes

1 small **sweet potato** (about 150 g/5½ oz), peeled and diced

1 small **carrot** (about 60 g/2¼ oz), peeled and thinly sliced

¼ small head **broccoli** (about 90 g/3¼ oz), cut into small florets

10 g/¼ oz **Cheddar cheese**, finely grated

Steam or boil the sweet potato in a saucepan over a medium heat for 5 minutes. Add the carrot and cook for a further 5 minutes, then add the broccoli and continue to cook for a further 5 minutes until all the vegetables are tender. Purée the vegetables with the cheese and 4 tablespoons of boiled water in a food processor, or using a hand blender, until smooth.

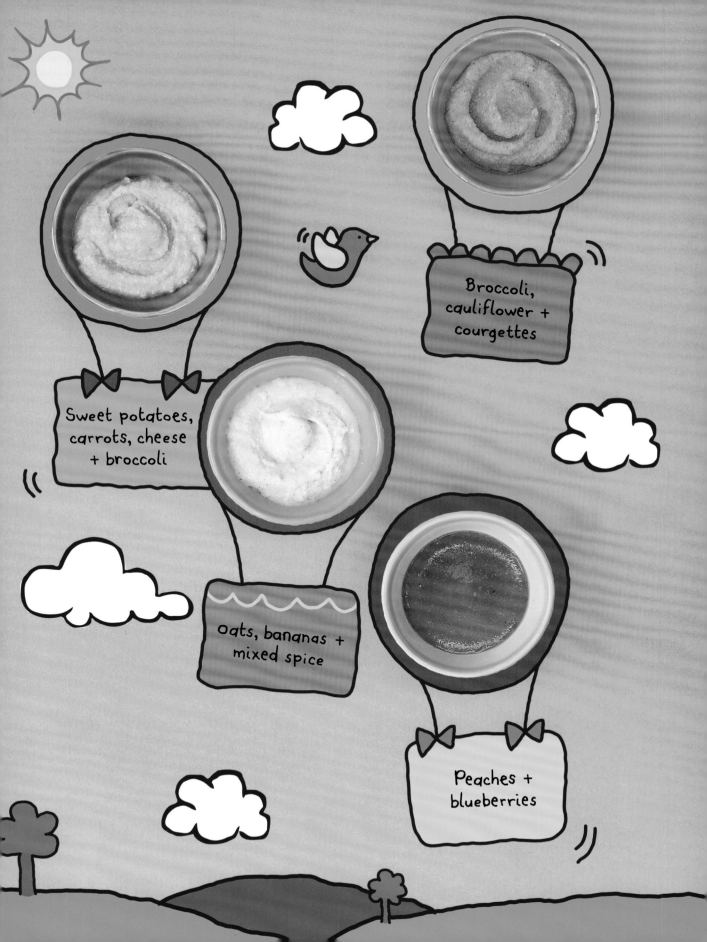

Broccoli, cauliflower + courgettes

Sweet potatoes, carrots, cheese + broccoli

oats, bananas + mixed spice

Peaches + blueberries

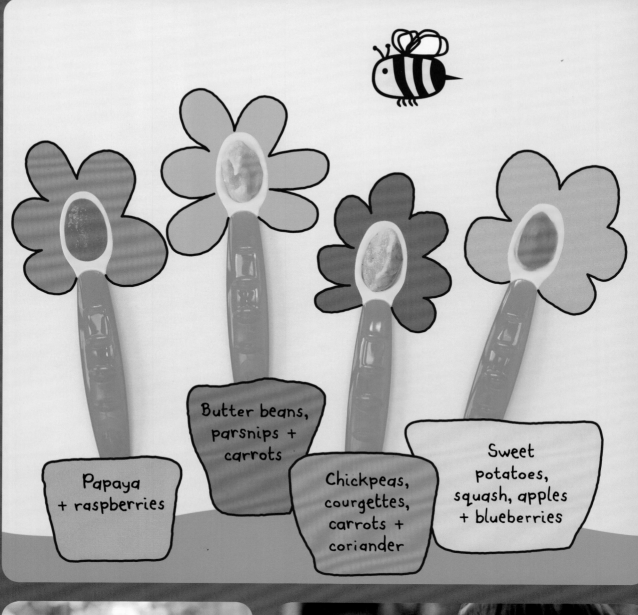

Papaya + raspberries

Butter beans, parsnips + carrots

Chickpeas, courgettes, carrots + coriander

Sweet potatoes, squash, apples + blueberries

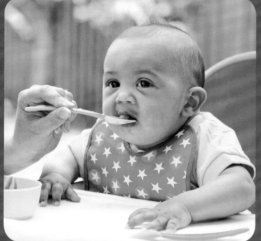
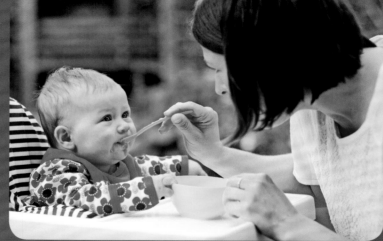

Papaya + raspberries

makes **6** ice cubes

prep **5** minutes

cook **no cook**

1 **papaya**, peeled, deseeded and diced

70 g/2½ oz **raspberries**

Purée the papaya and raspberries in a food processor, or using a hand blender, until smooth.

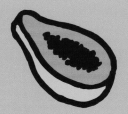

Butter beans, parsnips + carrots

makes **16** ice cubes

prep **5** minutes

cook **15** minutes

1 **parsnip** (about 150 g/5½ oz), peeled and diced

2 **carrots** (about 150 g/5½ oz), peeled and thinly sliced

100 g/3½ oz canned **butter beans** in water, drained and rinsed

Steam or boil the parsnip and carrots over a medium heat for 10–12 minutes until tender. Purée with the butter beans and 6 tablespoons boiled water in a food processor, or using a hand blender, until smooth.

Chickpeas, courgettes, carrots + coriander

makes **10** ice cubes

prep **5** minutes

cook **15** minutes

1 **carrot** (about 75 g/2½ oz), peeled and thinly sliced

1 small **courgette** (about 100 g/3½ oz), diced

10 **coriander** leaves

100 g/3½ oz canned **chickpeas** in water, drained and rinsed

Steam or boil the carrot and courgette in a saucepan over a medium heat for 8–10 minutes until they are tender. Add the coriander leaves and heat through. Purée with the chickpeas and 3–4 tablespoons of boiled water in a food processor, or using a hand blender, until smooth.

Sweet potatoes, squash, apples + blueberries

makes **13** ice cubes

prep **10** minutes

cook **15** minutes

⅓ **butternut squash** (about 150 g/5½ oz), peeled, deseeded and diced

1 small **sweet potato** (about 150 g/5½ oz), peeled and diced

3 small **eating apples**, peeled, cored and diced

25 g/1 oz **blueberries**

Steam or boil the squash and sweet potato in a saucepan over a medium heat for 10 minutes. Add the fruits and cook for a further 5 minutes until tender. Purée in a food processor, or using a hand blender, until smooth.

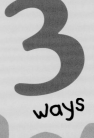

3 ways

Three ways with no-cook purées

Sometimes it helps to have a few quick and easy, no-cook purées up your sleeve for when time is short. All of these will rustle up in minutes and will make one hungry-baby portion. And just for fun, for each baby purée we've given a grown-up or toddler variation, too. Something for everyone!

Multi-melons + bananas

What you need

75 g/2½ oz **watermelon** flesh, deseeded and diced (you may need to sieve it if it's a bit stringy)

75 g/2½ oz **gala or cantaloupe melon** flesh, diced

1 small **banana**

1 tablespoon **natural Greek yogurt** (optional)

What to do

1. Put the melon and banana into a small bowl and whiz using a hand blender until completely smooth, then stir in the yogurt, if using.

Just for older ones

Double the recipe and take out your baby's portion. Pour 100 ml/3½ fl oz fresh apple juice into the remainder and whiz again. Serve over ice with a straw for a perfect summertime smoothie.

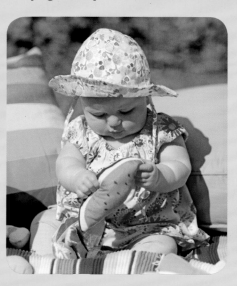

Our friends say...

'My baby and I were so often out and about, I created an on-the-go feeding survival kit! It had bowls with clip-top lids for purée, a little cool bag with squidgy freezer packs, and plenty of spoons in case any went on the floor!'

Peaches + cucumber cream

What you need

1 ripe **peach**, peeled and stoned, or ½ small can **peach slices in juice**

2.5 cm/1 inch **cucumber**, peeled and deseeded

1 tablespoon **natural Greek yogurt**

What to do

1. Chop the peach flesh and put it in a small bowl with the cucumber.

2. Whiz using a hand blender until completely smooth.

3. Add the Greek yogurt and stir to completely combine.

Just for older ones

Double the recipe and take out your baby's portion. In the remainder, add an extra tablespoon of yogurt and spoon into a ramekin. Sprinkle with granola and serve it up for a yummy breakfast or dessert.

Tangy kiwi + avocado

What you need

1 **kiwi fruit**

½ **avocado**

Just for older ones

If you want to use up the whole of the avocado, double the recipe, then take out what your baby needs. In the remainder add a squeeze of lemon juice and a splosh of olive oil, whiz it up and drizzle it over a green salad – delicious!

What to do

1. Peel the kiwi and chop the flesh. Put the flesh in a bowl with the avocado. Whiz using a hand blender until completely smooth.

2. Pass through a sieve to remove any remaining kiwi pips, if you like (although the pips are tiny and will be fine for babies over 7 months of age). Serve immediately.

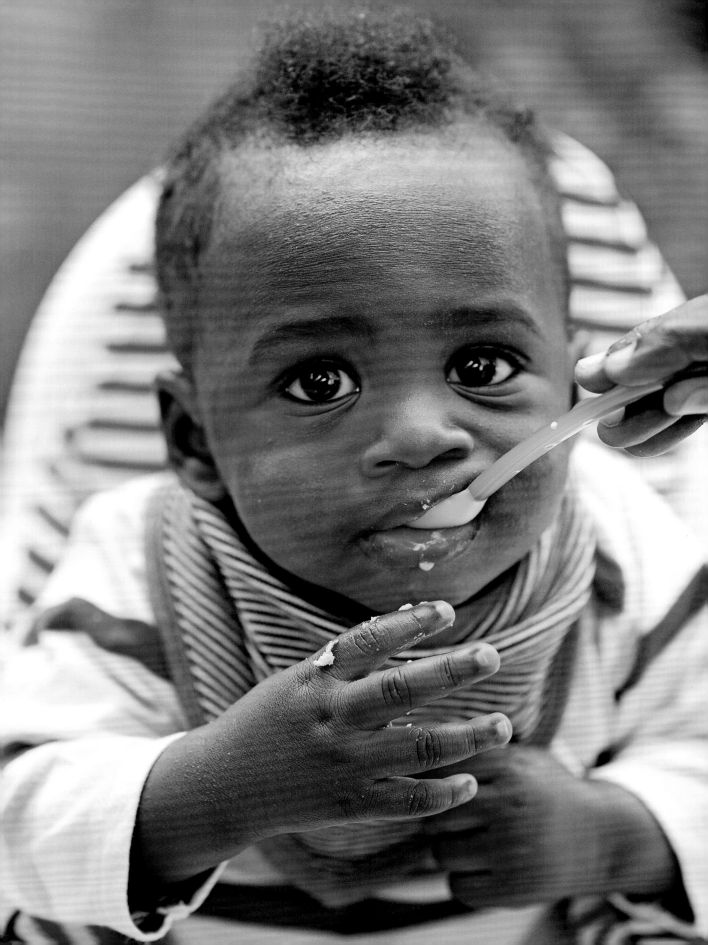

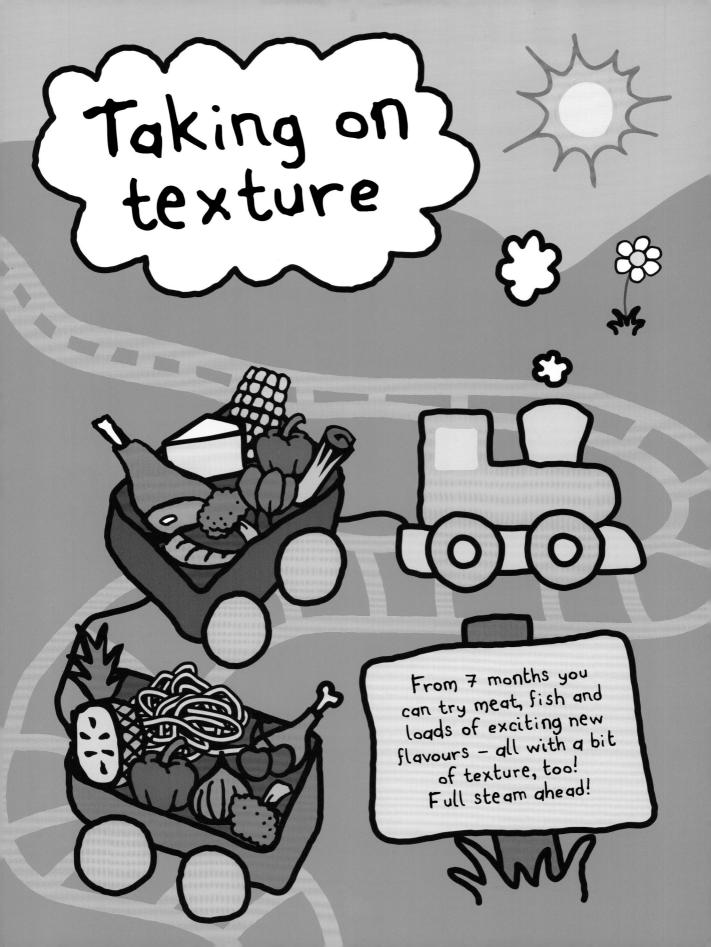

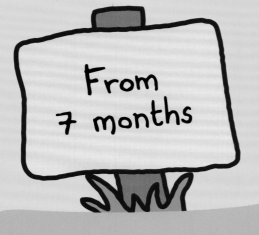

From
7 months

Your baby's digestive system is getting ready to tackle some protein foods, as well as meals with a little bit more texture. Many of the recipes in this chapter have been created as complete meals and introduce a more exciting blend of flavours and ingredients.

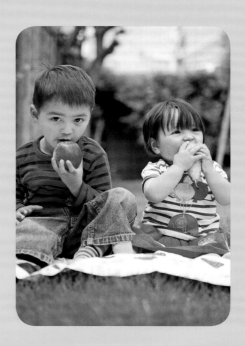

What to give

If you've been giving your baby a milk feed and then some purée, now is the time to start a mealtime with solids.

Continue to give 500 ml (17 fl oz) of milk a day as a drink, but your baby will also need essential nutrients, such as calcium, from food now. Introduce some meals made with milk to give calcium levels a boost for growing bones and teeth – cheesy pasta, creamy fish pie and rice pudding (pp.53, 71 and 75) are all good choices.

At 7 months your baby can start getting iron from red meat (beef and lamb), as well as pulses and all those lovely green veg. Meat, fish and pulses are also great for helping to develop immunity, as they contain iron and/or zinc.

Meat and fish (which are known as 'complete proteins') provide all the different protein building blocks your baby needs to grow. Dairy, pulses, nuts and seeds are also good protein sources, as are eggs (but cook them until both the white and yolk are solid).

Finally, babies need healthy omega-3 fats for their brain and eye development. Until now breastmilk or formula will have provided plenty, but the time has come for further supplies. Oily fish such as salmon (see p.63), sardines and pilchards are all good sources.

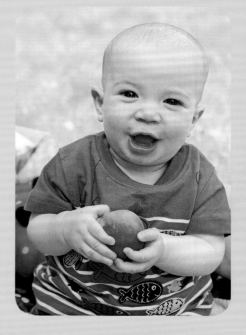

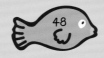

Tips on texture

Put away the blender and use a fork or a masher instead! Go for a texture of small, soft lumps in a thicker purée. Don't worry if you think your little one doesn't have enough teeth for the job – babies are clever and quickly learn to push little soft lumps against the roof of their mouth with their tongue, to squish before they swallow.

Avoid whole peas and sweetcorn, stringy or gristly meats, and hard pasta, though, as these can pose a choking risk. You may still need to purée foods with tougher skins, such as peppers, celery, green beans, pulses and onions.

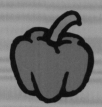

Nutritionist know-how

'Chewing not only makes food more interesting for babies, it helps to develop those little mouth muscles, encouraging speech development.'

Perfect timing

Your baby may be ready for 3 meals a day – breakfast, lunch and tea. You can give healthy snacks, but babies don't usually need them for nutrition reasons at this age (it's more about hand–eye coordination).

How much?

Depending on your little one's appetite, between 3 and 4 ice cubes of food per meal will be about the right amount. Remember to take your lead from your baby, who will tell you when enough's enough (see p.14). Of course, if you're met with tears when you take the spoon away, perhaps it's time for a bit more!

Tingling taste buds

Babies are very open-minded and experimental, so give some spices with a bit more oomph, such as cinnamon (try it with lamb; p.62) and cumin (with lentils; p.68). Introduce finger foods, too (see pp.152–7) – babies love feeling more in control of their eating and these are great for testing new flavours (and for developing hand–eye coordination).

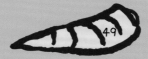

Little Bear's apricot porridge

makes **16** ice cubes prep **5** minutes cook **15** minutes

Tangy dried apricots in this warming porridge not only add a fruity twist, they also help boost your baby bear's iron stores.

What you need

40 g/1½ oz **porridge oats**

4 unsulphured, dark **dried apricots**, roughly chopped (see box, p.72)

¼ teaspoon **ground nutmeg**

300 ml/½ pint **baby's usual milk**, plus extra if needed

What to do

1. Place the oats, apricots, nutmeg and milk in a small saucepan and bring to the boil, then reduce the heat and simmer for 10 minutes, stirring frequently, or until the oats are cooked and the apricots are soft.

2. Using the back of a fork, mash the oat mixture until almost smooth, adding a little extra milk if necessary. Alternatively, purée in a food processor or using a hand blender.

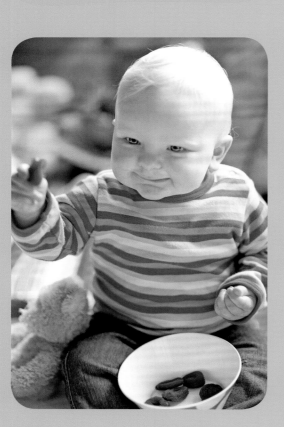

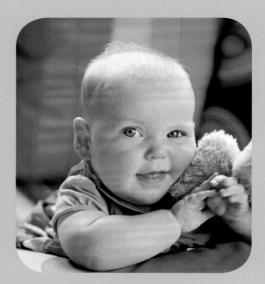

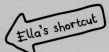
Ella's shortcut

You could try using a 70 g/ 2 oz pouch of Ella's Kitchen peaches, peaches, peaches as a yummy alternative to the dried apricots, if you prefer.

No-cook tuna + avocado mash

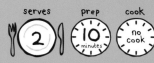

Perfect for when you've no time to cook, this tasty mash can be ready in minutes.

What you need

1 **tomato**

½ small **avocado**, stoned

A squeeze of **lemon juice**

2 tablespoons drained canned **tuna chunks** in spring water

3 tablespoons drained canned **haricot beans** in water, rinsed

Baby's usual milk (optional)

What to do

1. Place the tomato in a heatproof bowl and pour enough just-boiled water over to cover. Leave for 1–2 minutes, then carefully remove with a slotted spoon and peel off the skin. Halve the tomato, scoop out and discard the seeds, then finely chop the flesh.

2. Scoop out the avocado flesh into a bowl, squeeze over a little lemon juice and add the tomato, tuna and beans. Purée using a hand blender until almost smooth, adding a little milk if necessary.

Rough + smooth

Feed the senses

A whole avocado is brilliant for teaching opposites. Let your baby feel the bumpy skin – like a crocodile! Open it up for little fingers to poke the super-smooth flesh. Talk about the textures – rough and smooth all in one!

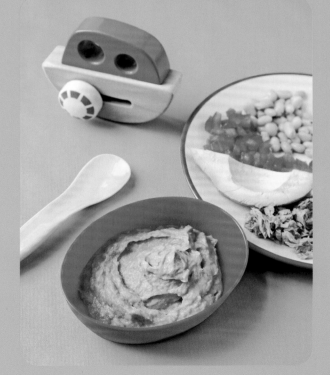

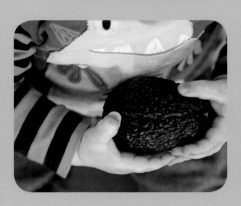

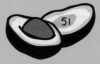

51

① Tropical pineapple zing

makes 18 ice cubes · prep 10 minutes · cook 15 minutes

What you need

25 g/1 oz **white basmati rice**

100 g/3½ oz **cottage cheese**

100 g/3½ oz **pineapple**, peeled, cored and very finely chopped

50 ml/2 fl oz **baby's usual milk**

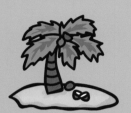

What to do

① Cook the rice in a small saucepan of boiling water according to the packet instructions until tender. Drain, then tip into a bowl.

② Add the cottage cheese, pineapple and milk, then using the back of a fork, mash together until almost smooth. Alternatively, purée in a food processor or using a hand blender.

② Cool summer soup

makes 21 ice cubes · prep 15 minutes · cook 5 minutes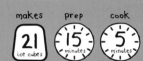

What you need

1 slice of **half-white, half-wholemeal bread**, crusts removed

6 tablespoons **baby's usual milk**, plus extra if needed

3 **tomatoes**

½ **red pepper**, cored, deseeded and cut into chunks

8 cm/3¼ inch piece of **cucumber**, peeled, deseeded and roughly chopped

150 g/5½ oz canned **butter beans** in water, drained and rinsed

A squeeze of **lemon juice**

A handful of **basil** leaves

What to do

① Place the bread in a shallow bowl, pour over the milk and leave to stand.

② Meanwhile, steam or boil the whole tomatoes and red pepper in a saucepan over a medium heat for 3 minutes until softened. When cool enough to handle, peel off the tomato skins and discard, then halve the tomatoes and remove the seeds.

③ Tear the bread into pieces, then purée with the tomatoes, red pepper, cucumber, butter beans, lemon juice and basil in a food processor, or using a hand blender, until almost smooth, adding extra milk or boiled water if necessary.

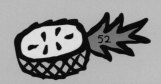

③ Supergreens cheese + chive pasta

makes 18 ice cubes · **prep** 5 minutes · **cook** 10 minutes

What you need

50 g/1¾ oz dried **orzo** or other dried **pasta**

3 **broccoli** florets, cut into pieces

25 g/1 oz **frozen petits pois**

½ teaspoon snipped **chives**

1 tablespoon **cream cheese**

5 tablespoons **baby's usual milk**

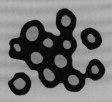

What to do

1. Cook the pasta in a saucepan of boiling water for 3 minutes, then add the broccoli and petits pois and cook for a further 4–5 minutes, or until everything is tender. Drain, reserving the cooking water.

2. Return the pasta, vegetables and 2 tablespoons of the reserved cooking water to the pan. Add the chives, cream cheese and milk and stir together.

3. Using the back of a fork, mash the pasta mixture until almost smooth. Alternatively, purée in a food processor or using a hand blender. To make the purée smoother, pass it through a sieve after blending.

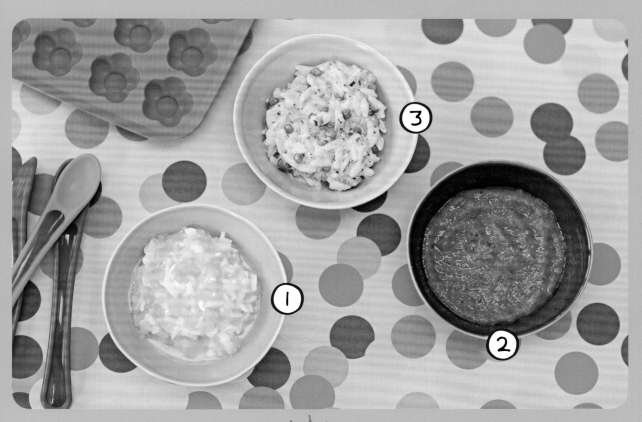

Roasty-red pesto chicken

makes
18 ice cubes

prep
15 minutes

cook
40 minutes

The juiciness of roast chicken gives a workout for little gums that are just learning to chew, and punchy pesto tingles tiny taste buds.

What you need

1 small **potato** (about 115 g/ 4 oz), peeled and thinly sliced into rounds

5 cm/2 inch piece of **leek**, white only, very thinly sliced

1 **tomato**, sliced into rounds

½ teaspoon **dried oregano**

1 teaspoon **olive oil**

1 teaspoon **red pesto** (see box, below)

1 skinless **chicken breast** (about 125 g/4½ oz)

Baby's usual milk (optional)

What to do

1. Preheat the oven to 200°C/400°F/Gas Mark 6. Place a large sheet of aluminium foil in a baking dish and arrange the potato in the middle in an even layer. Top with the leek and tomato, then sprinkle over the oregano and oil. Spoon the pesto over the chicken, then place on top of the tomato.

2. Gather up the edges of the foil and seal to make a parcel. Bake for 35–40 minutes until the potato is tender and the chicken is cooked through. Carefully open the parcel, remove the chicken and chop into four.

3. Whiz the remaining contents of the parcel with the chicken in a food processor, or using a hand blender, until finely chopped, adding a little milk if necessary.

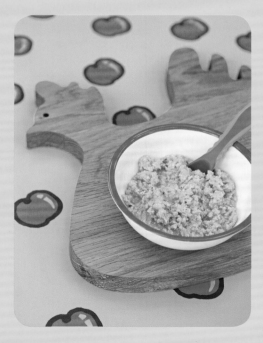

Perfect pesto

Homemade red pesto is super-easy! Heat 1 tablespoon of extra virgin olive oil in a nonstick frying pan, fry 2 chopped cloves of garlic and 100 g/3½ oz pine nuts for 2–3 minutes. Blitz 50 g/1¾ oz basil and 6 sun-dried tomatoes (drained and patted dry) in a food processor, then add the garlic mixture, 4 tablespoons of extra virgin olive oil, 50 g/1¾ oz Parmesan cheese and 100 ml/3½ fl oz water. Blitz again. (If you leave out the sun-dried tomato, the pesto is green!) Heat through before serving.

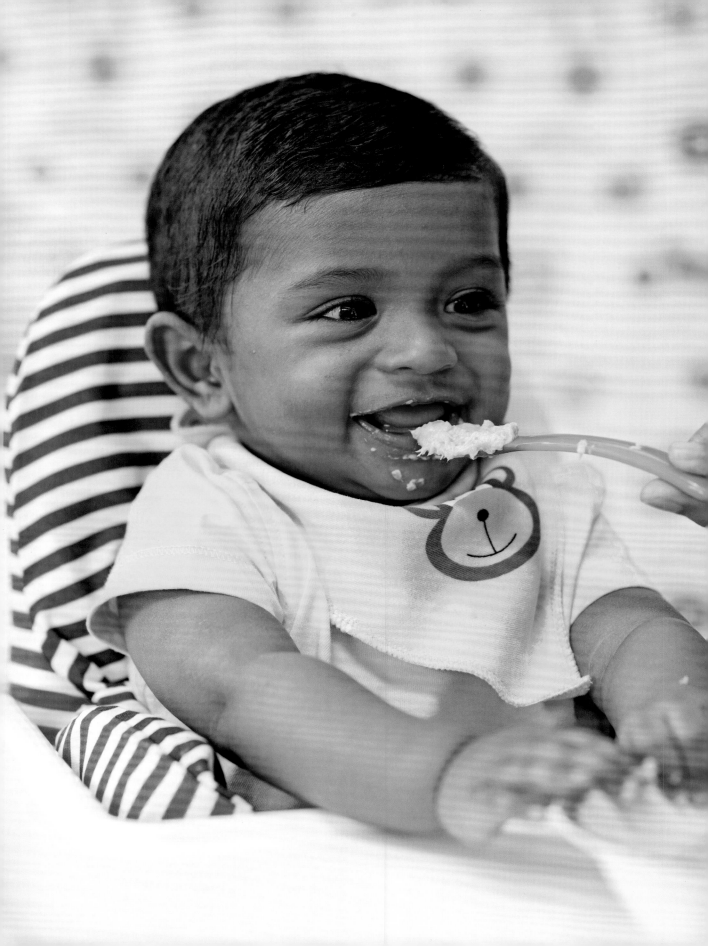

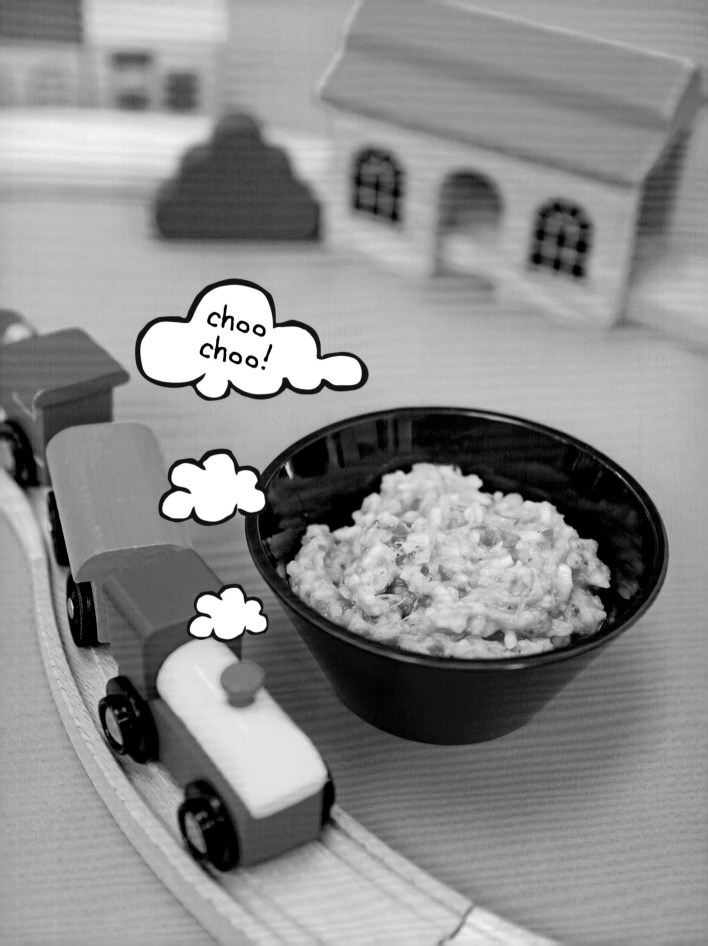

Tasty tomato-y fish + rice

makes **24** ice cubes · prep **10** minutes · cook **20** minutes

Tomatoes and green beans are full of vitamin C, which helps support little immune systems. This is a quick and easy dish – increase the quantities to feed the whole family, if you like.

What you need

25 g/1 oz **white basmati rice**

3 tablespoons drained canned **haricot beans** in water, rinsed

2 **green beans**, trimmed and chopped

2 teaspoons **olive oil**

115 g/4 oz skinless, boneless **white fish fillet**, such as haddock

175 ml/6 fl oz **passata** (sieved tomatoes)

½ teaspoon **dried oregano**

What to do

1. Cook the rice in a small saucepan of boiling water according to the packet instructions until tender, adding the haricot and green beans 8 minutes before the end of the cooking time.

2. Meanwhile, heat the oil in a nonstick frying pan over a medium heat and cook the fish for 10 minutes, turning once, until cooked through. Remove the fish with a spatula and flake into bite-sized pieces, taking care to remove any bones.

3. Drain the rice and beans, then place in a pan with the fish, passata and oregano. Cook over a low heat for 5 minutes, stirring frequently, until warmed through.

4. Using the back of a fork, mash the fish mixture until almost smooth, adding a little boiled water if necessary. Alternatively, purée in a food processor or using a hand blender.

Feed the senses

Super-shaker

Pop some uncooked rice in a clean plastic bottle and secure the lid. While you're rustling up this tasty dish, give the shaker to your baby to make some music for you to cook along to. Don't forget to dance! Lentils, crisped rice, and water are good shaker-fillers, too.

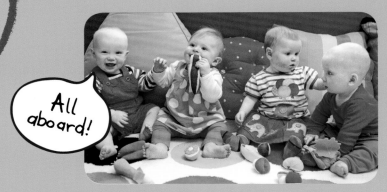

All aboard!

My first fish curry

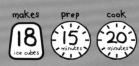

makes **18** ice cubes prep **15** minutes cook **20** minutes

Fish is a *reeeally* healthy source of protein to help your little taste explorer grow, and the exotic flavours in this dish make it perfect for baby's first curry night.

What you need

115 g/4 oz skinless, boneless **white fish fillet**, such as haddock

150 ml/¼ pint **baby's usual milk**, plus extra if needed

1 **lemongrass stalk** (optional)

25 g/1 oz **white basmati rice**

2 **broccoli** florets

1 teaspoon **mild curry powder**

2 tablespoons **coconut milk**

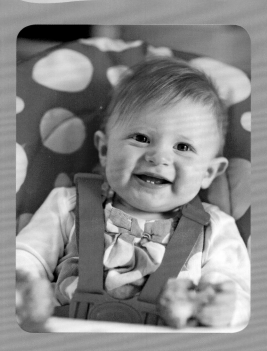

What to do

1. Place the fish in a small saucepan, cover with the milk and add the lemongrass (if using). Poach the fish over a medium–low heat for 12 minutes, or until cooked through. Reserving the milk, discard the lemongrass (if used) and lift out the fish with a spatula. Flake the fish into bite-sized pieces, taking care to remove any bones.

2. Meanwhile, cook the rice in a small saucepan of boiling water according to the packet instructions until tender. In a separate saucepan, steam or boil the broccoli over a medium heat for 6–8 minutes until tender. Remove and finely chop the florets, discarding the stalks.

3. Return the fish to the pan with the reserved milk. Drain the rice and add to the fish with the broccoli, curry powder and coconut milk. Stir over a low heat until combined and warmed through.

4. Using the back of a fork, mash the fish mixture until almost smooth, adding a little extra milk if necessary. Alternatively, purée in a food processor or using a hand blender.

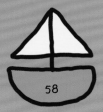

Warming veggie dhal

makes 18 ice cubes

prep 10 minutes

cook 20 minutes

This delicious dhal is made with red lentils, which are super-tasty *and* colourful, and also full of protein, helping your baby to grow big and strong.

What you need

50 g/1¾ oz dried **split red lentils**, rinsed

1 small **potato** (about 115 g/ 4 oz), peeled and diced

1 small **carrot** (about 60 g/ 2 oz), peeled and sliced

2 **cardamom pods**, split

1 teaspoon **mild curry powder**

2 tablespoons **coconut milk**

What to do

1. Place the lentils and potato in a small saucepan, cover with water and bring to the boil, then reduce the heat. Add the carrot and cardamom, part-cover with a lid and simmer for 13–15 minutes until everything is tender, skimming off any foam that rises to the surface. Drain, reserving the cooking water.

2. Return the lentils, potato and carrot to the pan, discarding the cardamom. Add 4 tablespoons of the reserved cooking water, the curry powder and coconut milk and stir until combined.

3. Using the back of a fork, mash the lentil mixture until almost smooth, adding a little extra reserved cooking water if necessary. Alternatively, purée in a food processor or using a hand blender.

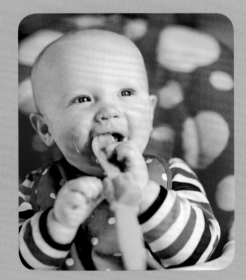

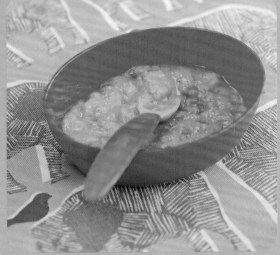

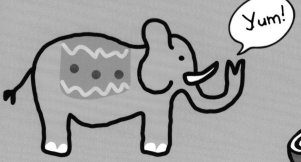

Yum!

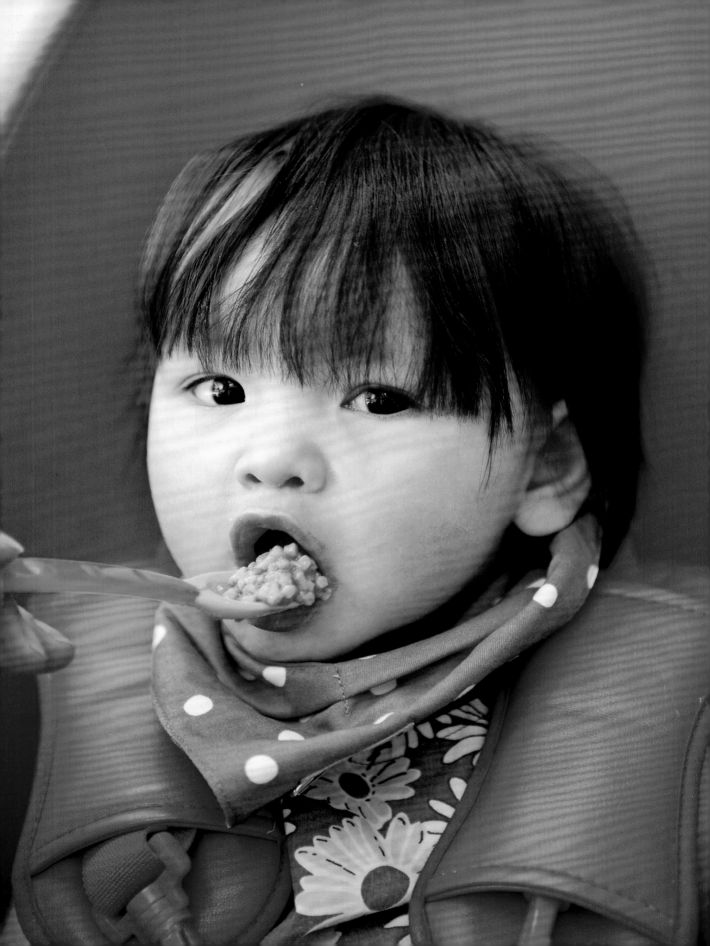

Super-simple spaghetti + sauce

We love this simple and speedy tomato sauce. It's really versatile, too – try adding puréed carrot or finely chopped spinach for different tasty flavours.

What you need

100 g/3½ oz dried **spaghetti**

2 teaspoons **olive oil**

1 **garlic** clove, crushed

200 ml/7 fl oz **passata** (sieved tomatoes)

½ teaspoon **dried oregano**, or a few **basil** leaves, chopped

2 tablespoons **crème fraîche**

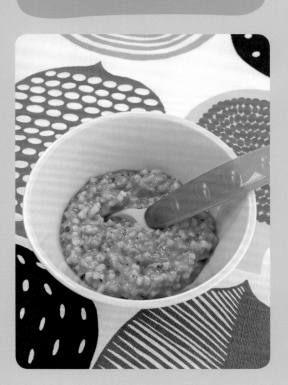

What to do

1. Cook the pasta in a saucepan of boiling water according to the packet instructions until tender.

2. Meanwhile, heat the oil in a small saucepan over a medium–low heat and cook the garlic for 1 minute, stirring, until softened. Add the passata and oregano or basil, part-cover the pan with a lid and simmer for 8 minutes until the sauce has reduced and thickened. Stir in the crème fraîche and heat through gently.

3. Drain the pasta, reserving the cooking water. Return the spaghetti to the pan, pour the tomato sauce over and turn the pasta until coated in the sauce.

4. Using the back of a fork, mash the pasta mixture until almost smooth, adding a little of the reserved cooking water if necessary. Alternatively, purée in a food processor or using a hand blender.

feed the senses

Herby water play

Babies love playing with water, so how about infusing it with herby scents? Pick off a few spare basil stalks and leaves and give your little one a small bowl of water (it might be best to do this outdoors or sitting on an oilcloth on the floor). Encourage your baby to swirl and squish the leaves and stalks through the water, mixing it up really well. Now, take a little cup and scoop out some of the water. Offer it to your baby to sniff. Can you smell the herb in the water? Try with some different fresh herbs – mint, sage and rosemary work a treat.

Sweet + spicy lamb + date couscous

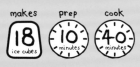

Delight tiny taste buds with this delicious combination of exciting new flavours.
The dates give a little burst of sweetness, while the cinnamon adds warming spice.

What you need

1 teaspoon **olive oil**

100 g/3½ oz **minced lamb**

1 small **garlic** clove, crushed

1 **carrot** (about 75 g/2½ oz), peeled and finely chopped

2 **pitted dried dates**, chopped

150 ml/¼ pint **passata** (sieved tomatoes)

½ teaspoon **ground cinnamon**

15 g/½ oz **couscous**

What to do

1) Heat the oil in a saucepan over a medium heat and cook the lamb mince for 5 minutes, breaking it up with the back of a fork, until browned all over.

2) Stir in the garlic, then add the carrot, dates, passata and cinnamon and bring almost to the boil. Reduce the heat, part-cover with a lid and simmer for 25 minutes until the sauce has reduced and thickened.

3) Meanwhile, place the couscous in a heatproof bowl and pour over enough just-boiled water to cover. Stir, cover with a plate and leave for 5 minutes until tender. Drain if necessary and add to the pan with the lamb. Cook for a further 5 minutes until tender, adding a splash of water if necessary.

4) Using the back of a fork, mash the lamb mixture until almost smooth, adding a little boiled water if necessary. Alternatively, purée in a food processor or using a hand blender.

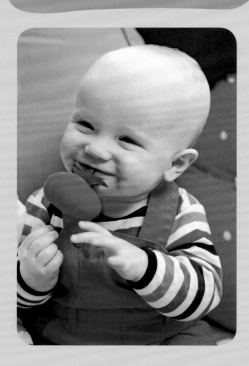

Keep smiling!

Smiley mealtimes keep babies happy about food. If your baby doesn't feel like eating, even if it's something *deeelicious*, that's okay. Don't look sad. Babies have hungry days and less hungry days – just like we do!

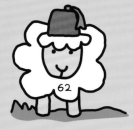

Wrapped + roasted salmon + beans

makes
18 ice cubes

prep
15 minutes

cook
35 minutes

Baking salmon in a little parcel keeps all the juiciness locked in, which means the salmon flakes will be super-soft for your baby's gums. Ground coriander adds a tasty twist.

What you need

1 small **potato** (about 115 g/4 oz), peeled and diced

115 g/4 oz skinless, boneless **salmon fillet**

½ teaspoon **ground coriander**

15 g/½ oz **unsalted butter**, cubed

2 **green beans**, trimmed and thinly sliced

5 tablespoons **baby's usual milk**, plus extra if needed

What to do

1. Preheat the oven to 190°C/375°F/Gas Mark 5. Place a large sheet of aluminium foil in a baking dish and arrange the potatoes in the middle in an even layer. Add 1 tablespoon of water, then top with the salmon. Sprinkle over the coriander and dot with the butter.

2. Gather up the edges of the foil and seal to make a parcel. Bake in the oven for 30 minutes until the fish and potato are cooked through.

3. Meanwhile, steam or boil the beans in a saucepan over a medium heat for 5 minutes until tender. Drain if necessary, then finely chop and return to the pan.

4. Open the foil parcel, tip the contents into the pan with the beans and add the milk. Heat through gently. Using the back of a fork, mash together until almost smooth, adding a little extra milk if necessary. Alternatively, purée in a food processor or using a hand blender.

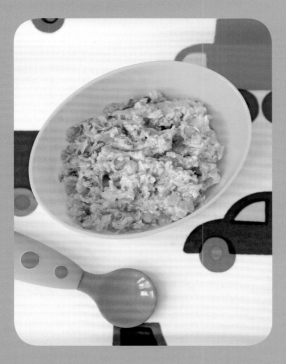

Our friends say...

'When I was breastfeeding, I ate lots of different spices so my little one got used to strong flavours in her milk feeds. It seemed to work – she's showing signs of becoming a really adventurous eater!'

oodles of noodles peanut-y chicken

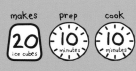

makes
20
ice cubes

prep
10
minutes

cook
10
minutes

This recipe introduces your baby to the tangy nuttiness of peanut butter, which is great for providing a protein boost for growing muscles and bones.

What you need

50 g/1¾ oz no-salt **egg noodles**

3 **broccoli** florets, cut into pieces

½ small **red pepper**, cored, deseeded and diced

2 teaspoons **sunflower oil**

1 skinless **chicken breast** (about 125 g/4½ oz), cut into chunks

5 tablespoons **baby's usual milk**, plus extra if needed

½ teaspoon **mild curry powder**

1–2 teaspoons no-salt, no-sugar **smooth peanut butter**

What to do

1. Bring a saucepan of water to the boil, add the noodles, broccoli and red pepper and cook over a medium heat for 4–5 minutes until tender. Drain, reserving the cooking water.

2. Meanwhile, heat the oil in a nonstick frying pan over a medium heat and stir-fry the chicken for 5 minutes until cooked through. Remove with a slotted spoon and finely chop.

3. Return the noodles, broccoli, red pepper and chicken to the saucepan with 4 tablespoons of the reserved cooking water, add the milk, curry powder and peanut butter and warm through.

4. Whiz the noodle mixture in a food processor, or using a hand blender, until finely chopped, adding a little extra milk if necessary.

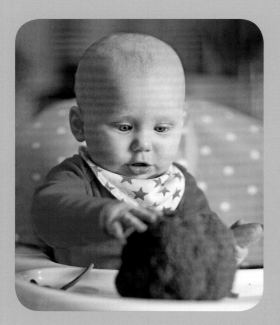

Mightily spicily!

Adding a little sprinkle of curry powder – or of spices such as paprika, cumin or coriander, and of lots of different herbs – is an easy way to send your baby on a taste adventure. Use just a touch here and there to tingle your baby's taste buds in a world of flavour.

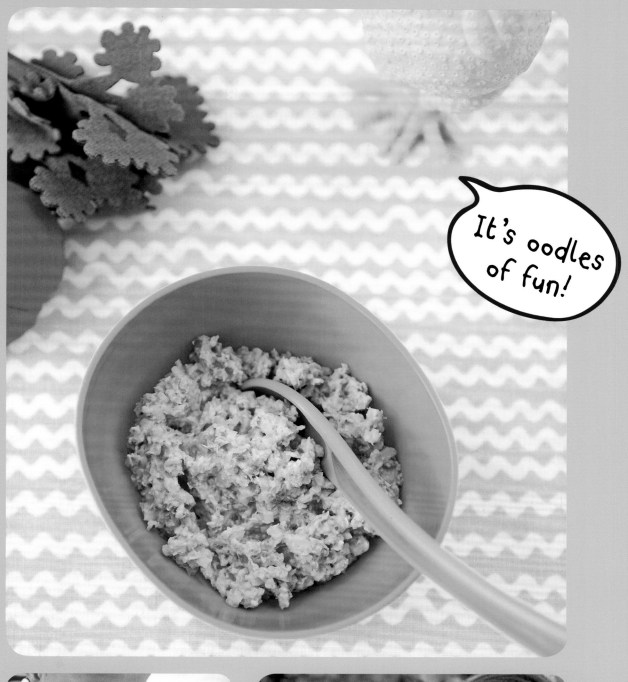

It's oodles of fun!

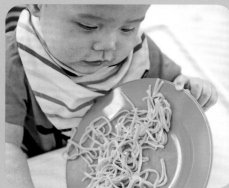

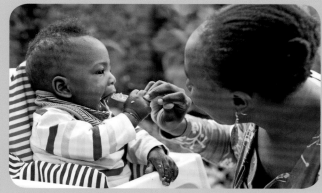

3 ways

Three ways with Ella's Kitchen Friends

We think the best weaning advice of all is passed on by word of mouth – from mums, dads, grannies and granddads, aunts and uncles, and from one friend to another. Some of those nuggets of wisdom might strike a chord and fire up an idea, and others might reassure, or make you smile and know that you aren't alone.

We've asked some of our Ella's Kitchen Friends for the best pieces of weaning advice others had given them. These are the ones we especially hope will inspire you to relax and enjoy this special time with your baby.

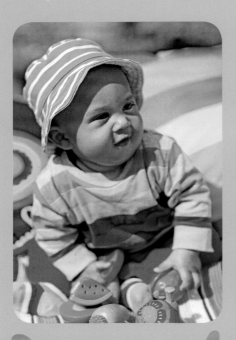

Take a look at our Weaning Adventure pull-out in the middle of the book. It's perfect for decorating the fridge and keeping lots of essential weaning info to hand!

Stick up lists

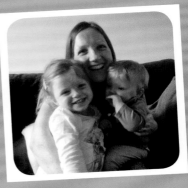

When I started weaning my little girl, the best piece of advice I think anyone ever gave me was to stick up a step-by-step list of when to introduce certain foods. It was a simple idea, but it made a big difference to us. It simplified the weaning process, which initially felt quite daunting. Once it was up, that list meant I could look on the fridge and plan my shopping with my baby in mind, knowing everything I bought for her was safe and providing the right nutrients. It also made it exciting when it was time to introduce something new – we'd celebrate with lots of smiles and cries of 'Well done!' Everyone was happy!

Saffron, mum to Allana (age 3) and Iris (age 8 months)

Look at a week

I used to think my little one was such a fussy eater and that he wasn't eating enough. Then, my health visitor told me I shouldn't think of his diet as something that happens over a day, but over the course of a week, or even a month. That was my lightbulb moment!

It sounds a bit grown-up, but I kept a food diary of everything he ate and the amount of time he spent breastfeeding every day for a month. It was amazing to see that some days he ate precious little in the way of food, but he certainly made up for it on others! Seeing everything written down made me realize that over a whole week, and then a whole month, he was eating perfectly well and getting everything he needed – he was just doing it his own special way!

Angie, mum to Reece (age 5) and Summer (age 2)

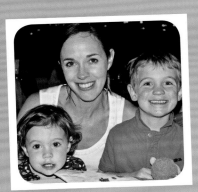

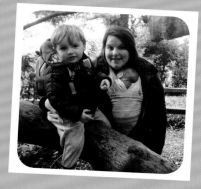

Turn the table

My baby boy was absolutely brilliant at eating in his high chair in the early days, but when he got a bit more mobile, he started objecting to sitting at the table. He wanted to eat on the move all the time!

My dad told me not to let it become a battle (eventually he'd sit where the rest of us were sitting), and to think of 'creative' tables around our home. At teatime, I took to laying out a picnic rug on the kitchen floor, with a few teddies, too; on warm days, we'd picnic in the garden. Teatimes were so much more relaxed this way that eventually, after only a couple of weeks and without him even really noticing, he was back in his high chair and eating at the table happily. Occasionally – even though he's now 3 – we still have an indoor picnic… just for fun!

Sophie, mum to Tristan (age 3) and Alice (age 10 months)

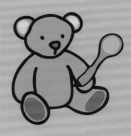

Very, very tasty veggie bake with lentils

makes
26
ice cubes

prep
10
minutes

cook
25
minutes

This dish is not only very, very tasty, it's very, very easy to make, too! It's crammed with veggies, and the cumin adds a smoky flavour for your little one to try.

What you need

1 small **sweet potato** (about 150 g/5¼ oz), peeled and cut into large bite-sized pieces

1 small **carrot** (about 60 g/2¼ oz), peeled and sliced

½ small **onion**, finely chopped

25 g/1 oz dried **split red lentils**, rinsed

150 ml/¼ pint canned **chopped tomatoes**

½ teaspoon **ground cumin**

2 hard-boiled **eggs**, yolks only, mashed

What to do

1) Place the sweet potato, carrot, onion and lentils in a saucepan, cover with water and bring to the boil. Reduce the heat, part-cover with a lid, and simmer for 15 minutes until tender, skimming off any foam that rises to the surface. Drain, reserving the cooking water.

2) Return the vegetables and lentils to the pan, add the tomatoes and cumin and stir in 2 tablespoons of the reserved cooking water. Simmer over a low heat for 5 minutes, then add the mashed egg yolks.

3) Using the back of a fork, mash the vegetable mixture until almost smooth, adding a little extra reserved cooking water if necessary. Alternatively, purée in a food processor or using a hand blender.

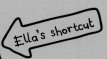
Ella's shortcut

Try using 2 x 70 g/2 oz pouches of Ella's Kitchen sweet potatoes, sweet potatoes in place of the sweet potato itself, and save on the chopping time!

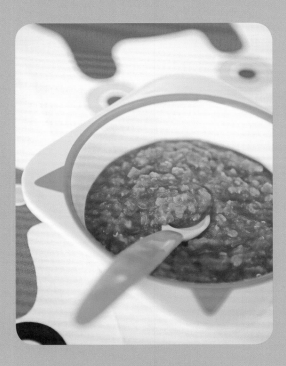

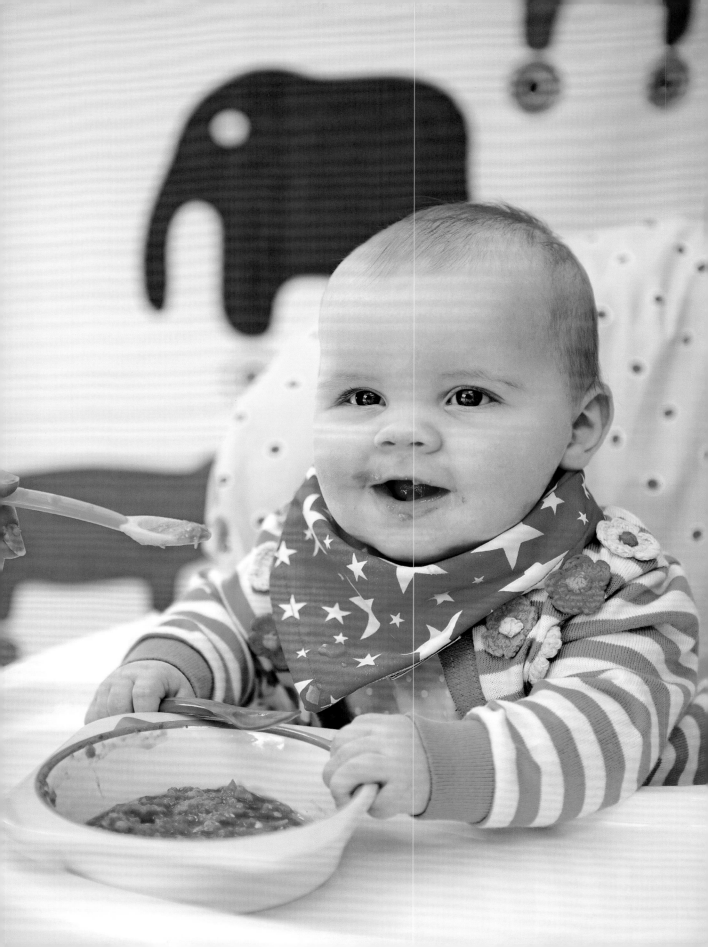

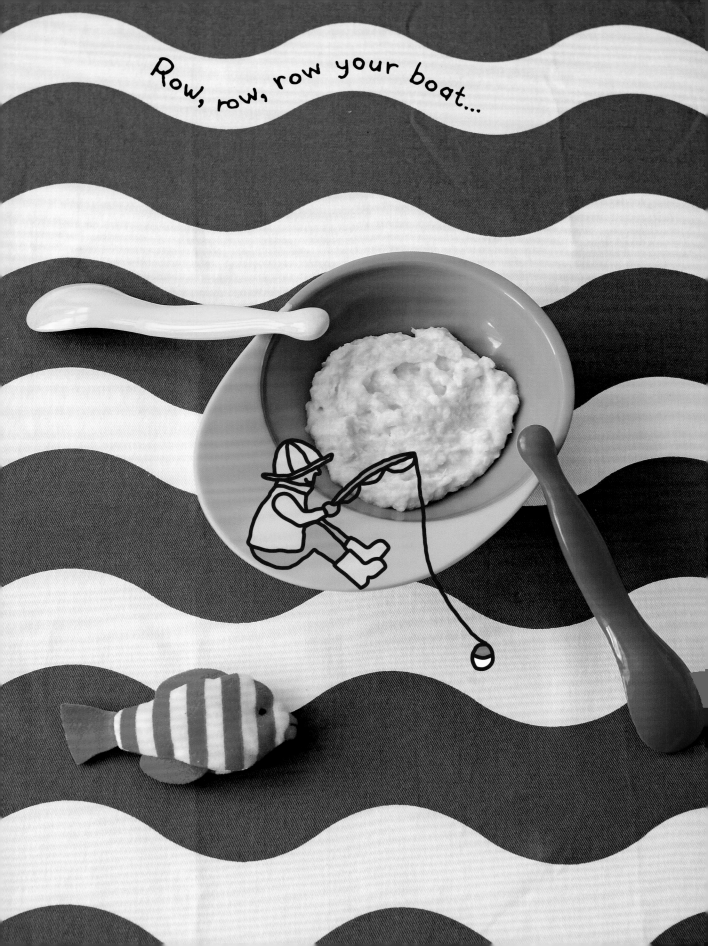

Row, row, row your boat...

Little fisherman's pie

This clever little pie uses crème fraîche to create a quick and easy sauce – brilliant for feeding hungry little fishermen and -women after a busy day at sea.

What you need

1 small **potato** (about 115 g/ 4 oz), peeled and quartered

1 **egg**

115 g/4 oz skinless, boneless **white fish fillet**, such as haddock

125 ml/4 fl oz **baby's usual milk**, plus extra if needed

1 **bay leaf**

½ small **leek** (about 50 g/1¾ oz), trimmed and thinly sliced

40 g/1½ oz no-salt, no-sugar canned **sweetcorn**, drained

2 tablespoons **crème fraîche**

Freezer-friendly

Mums often ask us if it's okay to freeze crème fraîche. Absolutely! This super-quick fish pie is perfect for popping in the freezer. Make two and save one for another day.

What to do

1. Place the potato in a small saucepan, cover with water and bring to the boil, then reduce the heat slightly and cook for 5 minutes. Add the whole egg to the pan and cook for a further 8 minutes until the egg is hard-boiled and the potato is tender. Drain, then cool the egg under cold running water.

2. Meanwhile, place the fish in a separate small saucepan and add the milk and bay leaf. Poach the fish over a medium–low heat for 12 minutes, or until cooked through. Reserving the milk, discard the bay leaf and remove the fish with a spatula. Flake the fish into bite-sized pieces, taking care to double check for any bones.

3. Steam or boil the leek in a saucepan over a medium heat for 6 minutes, then add the sweetcorn and cook for a further 2 minutes. Purée the vegetables in a food processor, or using a hand blender, until smooth.

4. Shell the egg, discard the white and chop the yolk. Place the yolk in the pan with the reserved milk and add the puréed vegetables, potato, fish and crème fraîche. Using the back of a fork, mash together until almost smooth, adding a little extra milk if necessary. Alternatively, purée in a food processor or using a hand blender.

Chick-chick chicken + apricot casserole

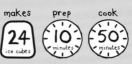

makes
24
ice cubes

prep
10
minutes

cook
50
minutes

This chicken recipe has a special ingredient – the pearl barley, which gives it a lovely, almost creamy texture and makes a nutritious alternative to rice, potatoes and pasta.

What you need

50 g/1¾ oz **pearl barley**, rinsed

3 unsulphured, dark **dried apricots**

2 teaspoons **olive oil**

100 g/3½ oz **minced chicken or turkey**

½ teaspoon **dried thyme**

A handful of **baby spinach leaves**, stalks removed and leaves finely shredded

250 ml/8 fl oz **baby's usual milk**, plus extra if needed

What to do

1. Place the barley in a small saucepan, cover with water and bring to the boil, then reduce the heat, part-cover with a lid and simmer for 30 minutes. Add the apricots and cook, part-covered, for a further 5 minutes until tender, then drain. Finely chop the apricots.

2. Meanwhile, heat the oil in a saucepan over a medium heat and cook the mince for 5 minutes, breaking it up with the back of a fork, until browned all over.

3. Add the thyme, spinach, milk, cooked barley and apricots to the mince and cook over a medium–low heat for 10 minutes, stirring frequently, until heated through and the mince is cooked.

4. Using the back of a fork, mash the mince mixture until almost smooth, adding a little extra milk if necessary. Alternatively, purée in a food processor or using a hand blender.

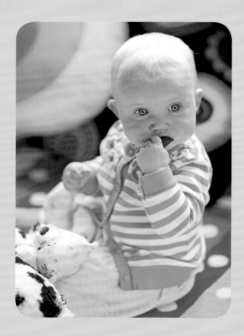

Best for tiny tums!

Always use unsulphured versions of dried fruits. Sulphur dioxide can sometimes cause allergies. Unsulphured dried apricots are brown in colour, so might not look as lovely, but they are just as yummy – and much healthier than the orange, sulphured kind.

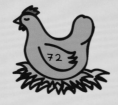

Full of beans pork + peppers

makes **26** ice cubes | prep **15** minutes | cook **35** minutes

The combination of soft pork and cannellini beans in this recipe is fantastic for introducing a bit of texture to little gums. Spinach and pepper contain vitamin C, which helps little ones release energy to keep them full of beans, too!

What you need

1 tablespoon **olive oil**

100 g/3½ oz lean **minced pork**

1 small **onion**, finely chopped

½ small **red pepper**, cored, deseeded and diced

1 **garlic** clove, crushed

1 teaspoon **dried thyme**

300 ml/½ pint **passata** (sieved tomatoes)

2 teaspoons **tomato purée**

2 **cloves**

100 g/3½ oz canned **cannellini beans** in water, drained and rinsed

25 g/1 oz **baby spinach leaves**, stalks removed and leaves shredded

What to do

1. Heat the oil in a saucepan over a medium heat and cook the mince for 5 minutes, breaking it up with the back of a fork, until browned all over. Remove with a slotted spoon and set aside.

2. Reduce the heat slightly, add the onion to the pan and cook for 5 minutes until softened, then stir in the red pepper, garlic and thyme and cook for a further 2 minutes, stirring frequently. Return the mince to the pan.

3. Stir in the passata, tomato purée, cloves, beans, spinach and 50 ml/2 fl oz water. Bring to the boil, then reduce the heat, part-cover with a lid and simmer for 20 minutes, stirring occasionally, until the mince is cooked through. Remove the cloves.

4. Using the back of a fork, mash the mince mixture until almost smooth, adding a little boiled water if necessary. Alternatively, purée in a food processor or using a hand blender.

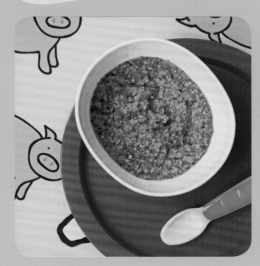

Sun-bleached splodges

We love a bit of mess at mealtimes, but how do you get the tomato-y blobs out of your little one's bib? We know! Pop it on a windowsill in the sunshine and the sun will bleach out the stains. Brilliant!

Rise + shine couscous with cherries + cinnamon

 makes **12** ice cubes

 prep **10** minutes

 cook **10** minutes

It's so important for little ones to experience a variety of different foods – and what better time to start than breakfast? (It's great as a pudding at other times, too.)

What you need

1 **eating apple**, peeled, cored and diced

50 g/1¾ oz **frozen pitted dark cherries**

150 ml/¼ pint **baby's usual milk**, plus 2 tablespoons

25 g/1 oz **couscous**

½ teaspoon **ground cinnamon**

Natural yogurt, to serve

What to do

1. Place the fruit and 100 ml/3½ fl oz water in a saucepan, cover with a lid and cook over a medium–low heat for 8 minutes until softened.

2. Meanwhile, pour the 150 ml/¼ pint milk into a small saucepan and warm over a medium heat. Stir in the couscous and cinnamon and reduce the heat to low. Cook for 5 minutes, stirring frequently, until the couscous is soft.

3. Transfer everything to a bowl. Using the back of a fork, mash together with the remaining milk. Or, purée in a food processor or using a hand blender. Serve with natural yogurt.

Creamy cheese + rosemary risotto

 makes **24** ice cubes

prep **10** minutes

 cook **25** minutes

Risotto is naturally soft and creamy, and this one oozes deliciousness.

What you need

75 g/2½ oz **risotto rice**

1 **garlic** clove, peeled and halved

1 teaspoon finely chopped **rosemary**

10 g/¼ oz **unsalted butter**

10 g/¼ oz **Parmesan cheese**, finely grated

80 g/2¾ oz **butternut squash**, peeled, deseeded and cubed

Baby's usual milk (optional)

What to do

1. Place the rice, garlic and rosemary in a saucepan, pour in 250 ml/8 fl oz boiling water and stir to combine. Cover and simmer over a low heat for 20–25 minutes, stirring frequently, until the rice is tender and water absorbed. Stir in the butter and Parmesan.

2. Meanwhile, steam or boil the squash over a medium heat for 15 minutes until tender. Mash until almost smooth, then stir into the rice. Mash again, adding a little milk if necessary. Or, purée in a food processor or using a hand blender.

Coconut + mango crush

makes 9 ice cubes · prep 5 minutes · cook no cook

Sunshine in a bowl – little ones won't be able to get enough of this speedy pudding. If you have a toddler, too, try freezing it into lollies!

What you need

85 g/3 oz ripe **mango** pieces

2 tablespoons **coconut milk**

2 tablespoons **baby's usual milk**

½ teaspoon **vanilla extract**

What to do

1. Place all the ingredients in a food processor or blender and blend until smooth and creamy.

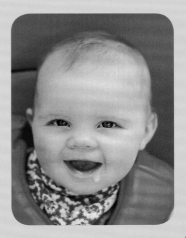

Spiced pear rice pud

makes 16 ice cubes · prep 5 minutes · cook 35 minutes

Pear is often a firm favourite with babies, and this creamy, warming rice pudding, made with risotto rice, is sure to delight.

What you need

200 ml/7 fl oz **baby's usual milk**, plus extra if needed

25 g/1 oz **risotto rice**

½ teaspoon **mixed spice**

1 ripe **pear**, peeled, cored and chopped

What to do

1. Pour the milk into a small saucepan and stir in the rice. Bring the milk almost to the boil, then reduce the heat, cover with a lid and simmer for 15 minutes, stirring frequently, until the rice starts to soften.

2. Add the mixed spice and pear, stir well and continue to cook, covered, for 15 minutes, stirring frequently to prevent the rice sticking to the bottom of the pan.

3. Using the back of a fork, mash the rice pudding until almost smooth, adding a little extra milk if necessary. Alternatively, purée in a food processor or using a hand blender.

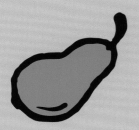

Frozen yogurt dots + fruity friends

Babies love getting their fingers messy in yogurty puddings, so how about this for a change? It's fruity yogurt frozen into slippery dots for little hands to hold. Brilliant!

Frozen yogurt dots

makes **8** ice cubes | prep **10** minutes + freezing

What you need

4 tablespoons **fruit purée** (see recipes, opposite)

4 tablespoons **thick natural yogurt**

What to do

1. Mix together the fruit purée and yogurt in a bowl.

2. Line a small baking sheet with baking parchment and place tablespoons of the yogurt mixture in individual piles on the paper. Place in the freezer for 2–3 hours until firm, then transfer to a freezer-proof bag and keep in the freezer for up to 1 month.

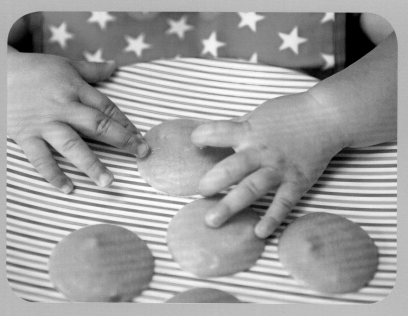

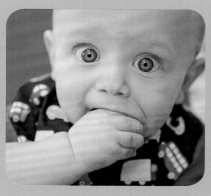

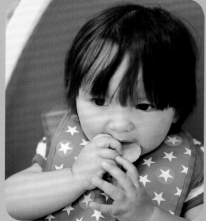

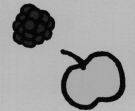

Tangy apricots + nutmeg

makes **6** ice cubes | prep **5** minutes | cook **15** minutes

75 g/2½ oz unsulphured, dark **dried apricots**, chopped

½ teaspoon **ground nutmeg**

Place the apricots and 200 ml/ 7 fl oz water in a small saucepan and bring almost to the boil. Reduce the heat, cover and simmer for 10 minutes until very tender. Stir in the nutmeg. Using the back of a fork, mash the apricots until smooth, adding extra boiled water if necessary.

Delicious dates + cinnamon

makes **6** ice cubes | prep **5** minutes | cook **15** minutes

75 g/2½ oz pitted **dried dates**, chopped

½ teaspoon **ground cinnamon**

Place the dates and 200 ml/ 7 fl oz water in a small saucepan and bring almost to the boil, then reduce the heat, cover with a lid and simmer for 10 minutes until very tender. Stir in the cinnamon. Using the back of a fork, mash the dates until smooth, adding extra boiled water if necessary.

Summer orchard fruits

makes **16** ice cubes | prep **10** minutes | cook **15** minutes

1 ripe **peach**

1 **eating apple**, peeled, cored and chopped

1 ripe **pear**, peeled, cored and chopped

Place the peach in a heatproof bowl and pour enough just-boiled water over to cover. Leave for 2–3 minutes, then carefully remove with a slotted spoon and peel off the skin. Slice the flesh away from the stone and set aside.

Meanwhile, place the apple, pear and 50 ml/ 2 fl oz water in a small saucepan and bring almost to the boil, then reduce the heat, cover with a lid and simmer for 8 minutes. Add the peach and cook for a further 2 minutes until the fruit is very soft. Using the back of a fork, mash until smooth.

Sunny berries

makes **9** ice cubes | prep **5** minutes | cook **no cook**

175 g/6 oz **frozen mixed summer berries**, defrosted

½ teaspoon **vanilla extract**

A pinch of freshly ground **black pepper** (optional)

Purée the berries and vanilla extract in a food processor, or using a hand blender, until smooth. Pass the purée through a sieve to remove any seeds and add a pinch of black pepper (if using).

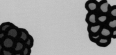

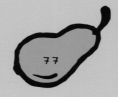

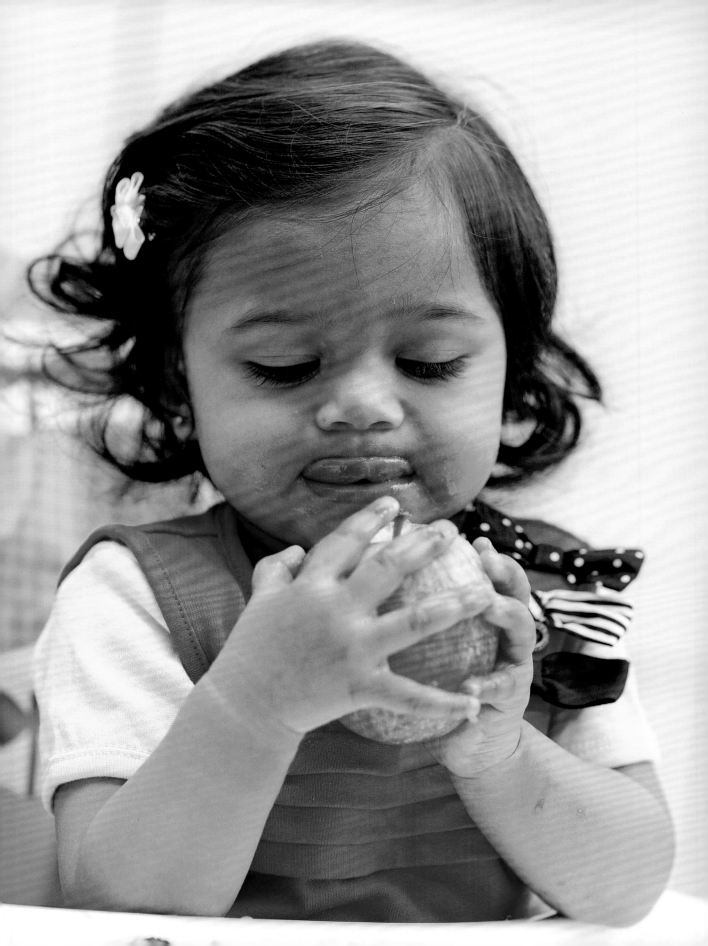

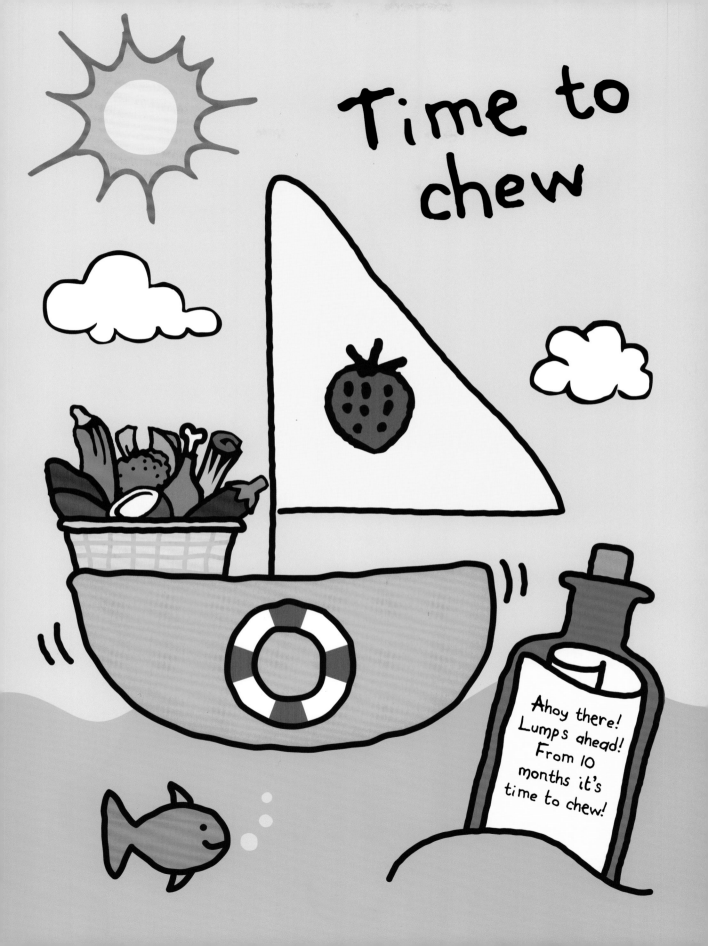

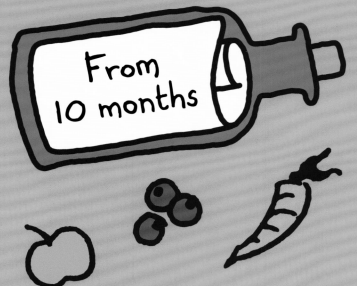

From 10 months

At 10 months old, babies often have a few first teeth – lumps and chunks are perfect for giving those new gnashers something to do. (If you haven't had any signs of teeth yet, don't worry – babies are brilliant at chewing soft chunks with just their gums.) Babies may now be starting to show some taste preferences, so all the recipes in this chapter help to keep the variety coming, many with stronger flavours, to encourage little ones to remain adventurous.

What to give

As little explorers become more mobile (some babies will be crawling and climbing; some may even be cruising), their energy requirements increase. Offer foods with good amounts of carbohydrate and protein for energy and keep healthy snacks on hand to pick up energy levels between meals. Try giving one mid-morning snack and one at mid-afternoon. Fruit chunks, yogurt, cheese, crackers and veggie sticks with dips (see pp.166–7) are all yummy options. And don't forget – babies still need around 500–600 ml (17 fl oz–1 pint) of their usual milk as a drink every day.

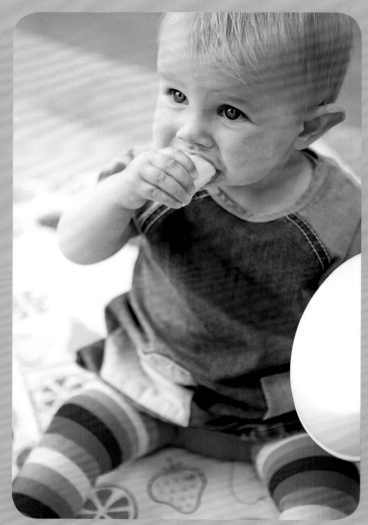

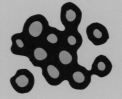

Tips on texture

You'll still need to mash or finely shred any meat and fish, but you can chop all other ingredients into small lumps now (not more than 1 cm/½ inch thick, though). At 10 months most babies can manage whole peas and sweetcorn kernels.

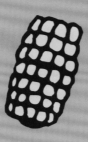

Make sure that lumps are held together in a thick purée, which helps keep everything moist and minimize the risk of choking. Avoid hard lumps in thin liquids and check that ingredients such as onion and beans aren't left with any fibrous bits or hard skin before you serve them up.

Nutritionist know-how

'If you're unsure how small to chop your little one's food, use the size of whole peas or blueberries as a guide.'

How much?

Your baby is ready for a heaped baby bowl of food at lunch and tea (and around a small bowl of porridge for breakfast). Here's our guide to portion size:

- 😊 A baby palm-sized amount of meat or fish
- 😊 A baby fist-sized amount of carbohydrate (pasta, potato, rice and so on)
- 😊 Between 1 and 2 portions of vegetables, where 1 portion is a baby handful

Some babies seem to eat a lot, others very little – that's perfectly normal. Babies' appetites vary a lot according to growth rates and how mobile they are. Also, sore, teething gums sometimes mean babies won't want to put anything in their mouths. Try not to worry – as long as your baby is growing and has plenty of energy, you're doing fine.

Tingling taste buds

Try combining sweet and savoury flavours – add fruit to a savoury dish (such as in Lovely Lamb with Mint + Pine Nuts; see p.91) or serving a zingy side sauce (try Mega Meatballs with Mango Sauce; p.105).

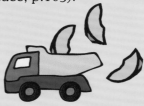

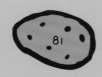

Super-soft oats + apples + seeds

serves **2** prep **10** minutes + overnight soaking cook no cook

You'll need to prepare this muesli the night before you intend to give it for breakfast – so that those delicious oats gets lots of time to soften and to soak up fruity goodness.

What you need

25 g/1 oz **porridge oats**

50 ml/2 fl oz **fresh apple juice**

1 tablespoon **sunflower seeds**

1 teaspoon **ground almonds**

3 tablespoons **cooked apple flesh** or **apple purée**

3 tablespoons **natural yogurt** or **baby's usual milk**

A large pinch of **ground cinnamon**

What to do

1) Place the oats in a bowl. Pour over the apple juice and 50 ml/2 fl oz water. Stir, cover with clingfilm and soak overnight in the fridge.

2) The next morning, grind the sunflower seeds to a coarse powder with a pestle and mortar, then stir into the oats with the ground almonds, cooked apple or apple purée, the yogurt or milk and the cinnamon. Using the back of a fork, mash the muesli to a coarse purée, adding more yogurt if necessary.

Cheeky beans + baked eggs

serves **2–3** prep **5** minutes cook **15** minutes

Eggs, beans and even carrots – this is a cooked breakfast Ella's Kitchen-style!

What you need

1 **carrot**, peeled and thinly sliced

75 g/2½ oz canned **haricot beans** in water, drained

2 tablespoons **tomato purée**

10 g/¼ oz **unsalted butter**

2 hard-boiled **eggs**, yolks only, mashed

Toasted **bread**, cut into fingers, to serve

What to do

1) Steam or boil the carrot over a medium heat for 10–12 minutes until tender. Purée the carrot with 2 tablespoons of boiled water in a food processor, or using a hand blender, until smooth.

2) Meanwhile, place the beans, tomato purée and butter in a separate small saucepan and cook gently for 5 minutes, stirring frequently, until softened. Add the puréed carrot, egg yolks and 4 tablespoons of boiled water, stir and heat through. Mash to a coarse purée, adding a little extra water if necessary. Serve with toast fingers.

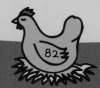

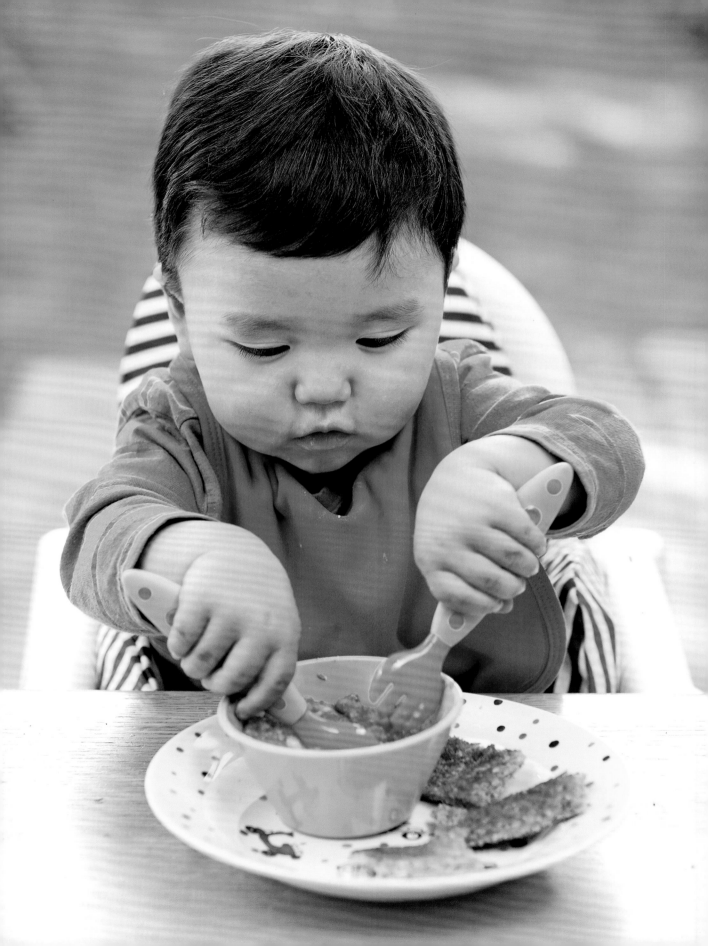

Shake-it-up scrambled eggs

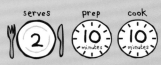

serves 2 | prep 10 minutes | cook 10 minutes

We've crammed loads of extras into these scrambled eggs to make them especially delicious. Our little taste tester at our photoshoot gave them a massive cheer!

What you need

10 g/¼ oz **unsalted butter**

1 **tomato**, deseeded and diced

1 **spring onion**, very finely chopped

2 tablespoons no-salt, no-sugar canned **sweetcorn**, drained

A large pinch of **Chinese 5-spice**

2 **eggs**, lightly beaten

2 tablespoons **whole milk**

Small **pitta bread**, warmed and cut into fingers, to serve

What to do

1. Heat half the butter in a small saucepan over a medium–low heat and cook the tomato, spring onion and sweetcorn for 5 minutes, stirring frequently, until softened. Stir in the 5-spice.

2. Beat together the eggs and milk in a small bowl or jug.

3. Add the remaining butter to the pan and when melted pour in the egg mixture. Cook over a low heat, stirring and folding the eggs continuously until scrambled. Serve with fingers of pitta bread.

Eggy variations

Instead of the sweetcorn and Chinese 5-spice, you could add some cooked peas and a little fresh thyme or basil.

Or, shred a few baby spinach leaves and cook with the tomato and spring onion (leave out the sweetcorn), and stir in a pinch of mild curry powder.

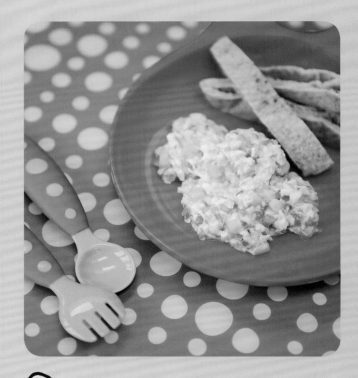

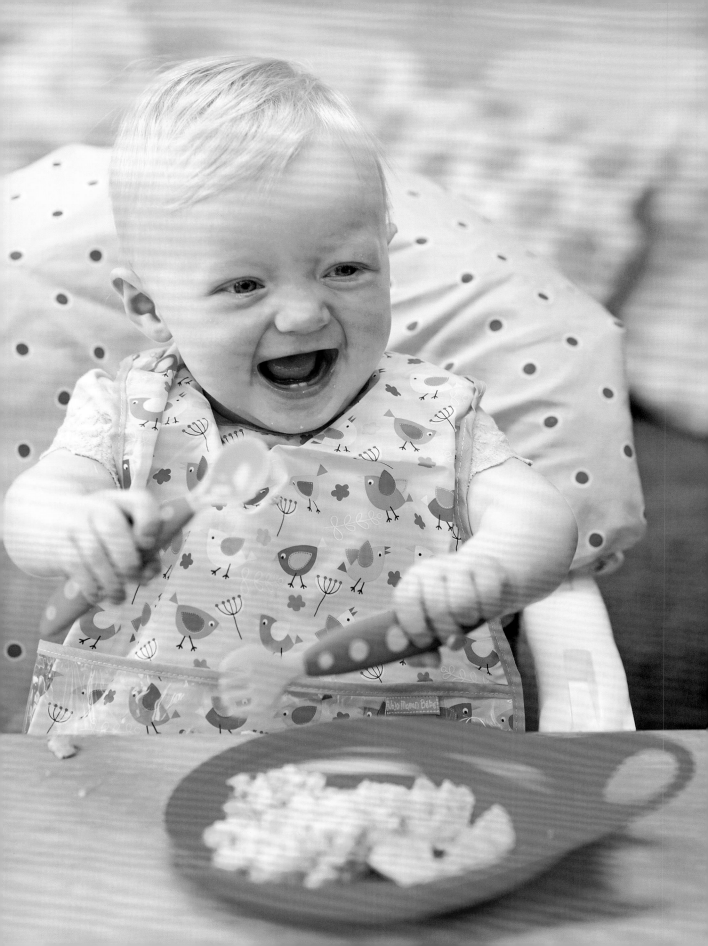

Buttery leek + chicken pie

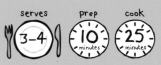

We've topped this chicken pie with slices of new potato and packed it with yummy leek and scrummy sweetcorn – to give you a hearty meal for your baby.

What you need

200 g/7 oz **new potatoes**, scrubbed, and halved if large

15 g/½ oz **unsalted butter**

1 skinless **chicken breast** (about 125 g/4½ oz), cut into bite-sized pieces

1 **leek**, trimmed, cleaned and finely chopped

6 tablespoons drained no-salt, no-sugar canned **sweetcorn**

1 heaped teaspoon **cornflour**

150 ml/¼ pint **whole milk**

½ teaspoon **English mustard**

½ teaspoon **dried thyme**

A little **olive oil**, for brushing

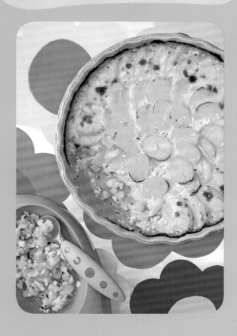

What to do

1. Cook the potatoes in a saucepan of boiling water for 10–15 minutes until tender. Drain and leave to dry and cool slightly, then peel off the skins and cut into thin slices.

2. Meanwhile, melt the butter in a saucepan over a medium heat and cook the chicken for 5 minutes until browned all over and cooked through. Remove with a slotted spoon and set aside. Add the leek to the pan and cook for 3 minutes until tender. Stir in the sweetcorn and heat through, then return the chicken to the pan.

3. Mix the cornflour into a little of the milk. Pour the remaining milk into the pan with the mustard and thyme and heat over a medium–low heat. Stir in the cornflour mixture and cook gently for 5 minutes, stirring, until the sauce has thickened.

4. Preheat the grill to medium–high. Spoon the chicken mixture into a small ovenproof dish and top evenly with the sliced potatoes. Brush the top with a little oil and grill for 10 minutes, or until slightly golden.

5. Using the back of the fork, mash the pie to a coarse purée, adding a little boiled water if necessary. Alternatively, finely chop.

 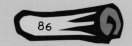

Pop-out mini-tortilla muffins

serves 8 | prep 15 minutes | cook 30 minutes

Baking mini tortillas in a muffin tin is just so easy! These are packed full of veg and are great mashed up, or left whole for little hands to hold.

What you need

Unsalted butter or **olive oil**, for greasing

1 **potato** (about 200 g/7 oz), peeled and quartered

60 g/2¼ oz **frozen petits pois**

½ **red pepper**, cored, deseeded and cut into small dice

6 **eggs**, lightly beaten

2 **spring onions**, finely chopped

40 g/1½ oz **Parmesan cheese**, finely grated

Freshly ground **black pepper**

Broccoli and **wholemeal rolls**, to serve

What to do

1. Preheat the oven to 180°C/350°F/Gas Mark 4. Grease 8 holes of a deep muffin tin.

2. Steam or boil the potato in a saucepan over a medium heat for 8 minutes until almost tender. Add the petits pois and red pepper and cook for a further 5 minutes, or until all the vegetables are tender.

3. Meanwhile, beat the eggs in a large bowl. Stir in the spring onions and Parmesan and season with a little pepper.

4. Drain the vegetables if necessary, then leave to cool slightly. Cut the potatoes into cubes, then stir them into the egg mixture with the peas and red pepper.

5. Ladle the egg mixture evenly into the prepared muffin tin. Bake in the oven for 15 minutes until the tortillas are cooked through. Leave to cool slightly before serving with broccoli and bread rolls.

Lunchbox lovelies

These mini tortillas are perfect for lunch on the go, and for toddler lunchboxes, too. Once they're cool, the tortillas will keep in the fridge in an airtight container for up to 3 days.

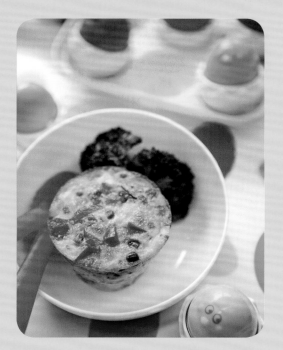

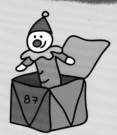

87

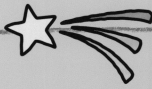

Shooting stars sardine pasta

serves **2–3** · prep **10** minutes · cook **15** minutes

Sardines are loaded with essential fatty acids, making them a superstar ingredient for developing little brains and eyes!

What you need

60 g/2¼ oz small **star-shaped dried pasta**

A large handful of **baby spinach leaves**, stalks removed and leaves finely chopped

120 g/4¼ oz can **sardines** in water, drained and large bones removed

2 teaspoons **extra virgin olive oil**

2 **tomatoes**, deseeded and diced

2 tablespoons **tomato purée**

1 tablespoon chopped **basil** leaves

What to do

1. Cook the pasta in a saucepan of boiling water according to the packet instructions, until tender, adding the spinach 2 minutes before the end of the cooking time. Drain, reserving the cooking water.

2. Meanwhile, mash the sardines in a bowl.

3. Heat the oil in a small saucepan over a medium–low heat and cook the tomatoes for 2 minutes until softened. Add the tomato purée, basil, sardines, cooked pasta and spinach and 4 tablespoons of the reserved cooking water and heat for 3 minutes, stirring frequently.

4. Using the back of a fork, mash the pasta mixture to a coarse purée, adding a little boiled water if necessary. Or, finely chop.

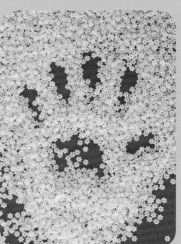

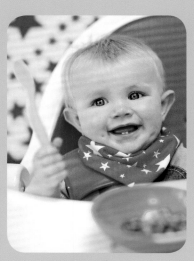

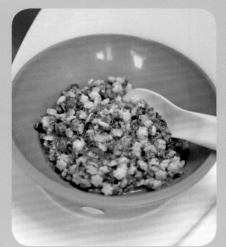

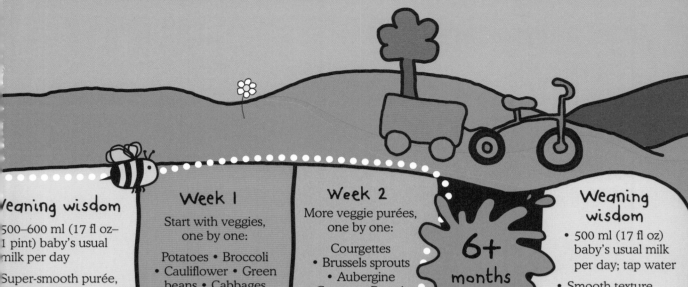

Weaning wisdom

500–600 ml (17 fl oz–1 pint) baby's usual milk per day

Super-smooth purée, like runny honey

2–3 teaspoons, once a day

Week 1

Start with veggies, one by one:

Potatoes • Broccoli • Cauliflower • Green beans • Cabbages • Avocado • Peas

Week 2

More veggie purées, one by one:

Courgettes • Brussels sprouts • Aubergine • Carrots • Parsnips • Butternut squash • Swede

6+ months

Weaning wisdom

• 500 ml (17 fl oz) baby's usual milk per day; tap water

• Smooth texture, but slightly thicker

• 1–2 ice cubes, twice a day

Veggies + fruit

All veg + fruit are good, and in purée combos, too

Weaning wisdom

• 500 ml (17 fl oz) baby's usual milk per day; tap water; well-diluted fresh juice

• Mashed-up, very soft texture with very small, soft lumps

• 3–4 ice cubes, 3 times a day

7+ months

Grains + pulses

Try purées with:

Cereal foods (such as pasta) • Rice • Lentils • Chickpeas • Beans, including soya beans

Dairy + eggs

Try purées with:

Natural full-fat yogurt, fromage frais or crème fraîche • Cooked full-fat cow's, sheep's or goat's milk • Pasteurized cheese • Well-cooked eggs

...wisdom

... fl oz) full-fat ... daily; tap water ... 7+ months

... ized pieces

... wl 3 times ... nacks

Dairy + eggs

Try meals made with:

Well-cooked unpasteurized soft or blue cheese • Runny eggs

Other yummy foods

Now your baby can try a little honey

One last thing...

Your baby can eat anything now, but some foods still pose a choking risk. Avoid:

Whole nuts • Whole grapes + other whole fruits with shiny skins

Finally, always avoid adding sugar or salt to your little one's meals.

Step-by-step weaning adventure

Hooray! It's time to start your baby's weaning journey. Follow the path, one step at a time, all the way to family mealtimes!

Very first tastes
First 2 weeks

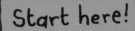

Start here!

Veggie tastes and baby's milk are all your baby needs for now. Avoid the following:

Dairy + eggs • Grains + pulses • Poultry + meat • Fish + shellfish • Nuts + seeds • Other foods: celeriac, celery, honey

Nuts + seeds

Try mashed-up meals with:

Smooth peanut butter • Finely ground nuts • Finely ground seeds

Fish + shellfish

Try mashed-up meals with:

Salmon + white fish • Canned tuna • Sardines + mackerel • Well-cooked prawns

Poultry + meat

Try mashed-up meals with:

Soft, lean poultry • Soft, lean meat

Dairy + eggs

Now your baby can try mashed-up meals with cooked unpasteurized hard cheese

10+ months

Weaning wisdom

• Drinks as 7+ months

• Soft pea-sized lumps + chunks in a thick purée

• Heaped bowl 3 times a day + 2 snacks

Nuts + seeds

Try chunkier meals with:

Finely chopped nuts • Finely chopped seeds

Other yummy foods

Liven things up with stronger spices, such as ginger

12+ months

Weaning

• 500 ml (17 cow's milk + juice as

• Baby bite-s

• Heaped bo a day + 2 s

open me
to find your
pull-out weaning
planner!

Open me
to find your
pull-out weaning
wall chart!

wall chart

ll your favourite foody memories

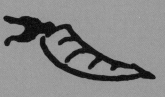

rite fruits

....
....
....

I ate my first
finger food on...

When I was 10 months,
I loved eating...

1 ....
2 ....
3 ....
4 ....
5 ....

When I was 6 months,
I loved eating...

1 ....
2 ....
3 ....
4 ....
5 ....

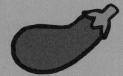

ike to share
me with...

When I was 7 months,
I loved eating...

1 ....
2 ....
3 ....
4 ....
5 ....

Now I'm one year old,
I love eating...

1 ....
2 ....
3 ....
4 ....
5 ....
6 ....
7 ....

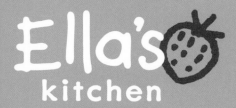 **Ella's kitchen** **My weaning v**

Stick up this wall chart and fill it in with a

Stick a picture of you with a messy, foody face here

I took my very first yummy mouthful on...

My very first purée was...

My favou

1 ....
2 ....
3 ....
4 ....
5 ....

My first chompy tooth popped through on...

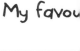

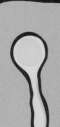 I did some scooping with my very own spoon on...

My favourite veggies

1 ....
2 ....
3 ....
4 ....
5 ....

I most
teati

 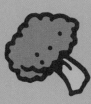

Super-scrummy salmon risotto

serves **4**   prep **15** minutes   cook **45** minutes

The thyme in this recipe gives our creamy salmon risotto an exciting flavour twist, while the soft salmon is perfect for new little teeth to practise their chomping skills.

What you need

175 g/6 oz skinless, boneless **salmon fillet**

100 ml/3½ fl oz **whole milk**

2 teaspoons **olive oil**

1 small **onion**, finely chopped

75 g/2½ oz **risotto rice**

350 ml/12 fl oz **vegetable stock**

40 g/1½ oz **frozen petits pois**

1 teaspoon **dried thyme**

2 tablespoons chopped **flat-leaf parsley** (optional)

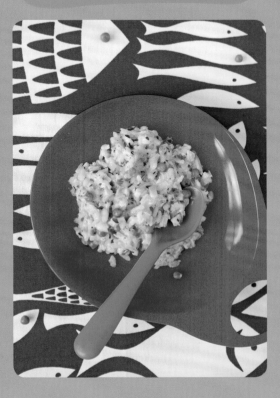

What to do

1. Place the salmon in a small saucepan and cover with the milk. Poach over a medium–low heat for 10 minutes, or until cooked through. Reserving the milk, remove the fish with a spatula. Flake the fish into bite-sized pieces, taking care to remove any bones.

2. Meanwhile, heat the oil in a saucepan over a medium heat. Add the onion, part-cover with a lid and cook for 8 minutes, stirring frequently, until softened. Add the rice and stir until combined with the onions. Pour in the stock and cook for 25 minutes, stirring frequently, until the rice is tender.

3. Add the petits pois and thyme and cook for a further 3 minutes, then add the cooked salmon and half the reserved milk and heat through, adding more of the milk if necessary. Stir in the parsley (if using), cover with a lid and leave to stand for 3 minutes.

4. Using the back of a fork, mash the rice mixture to a coarse purée, adding more of the reserved milk if necessary. Alternatively, finely chop.

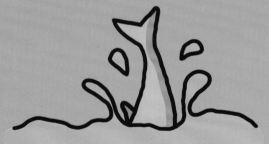

Veggie feast mac + cheese

There are so many different ways to make mac + cheese, but we think this one is by far the best. Courgettes and petits pois provide veggie goodness, while a little bit of mustard gives a tasty kick.

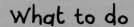

What you need

60 g/2¼ oz dried **macaroni**

20 g/¾ oz **frozen petits pois**

1 small **courgette**, grated

10 g/½ oz **unsalted butter**

2 teaspoons **plain flour**

150 ml/¼ pint **whole milk**, warmed, plus extra if needed

½ teaspoon **Dijon mustard**

30 g/1 oz **Cheddar cheese**, grated

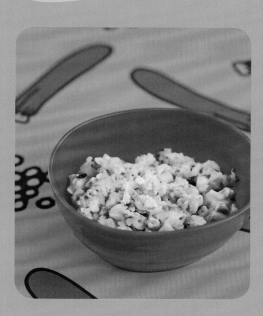

What to do

1. Preheat the oven to 180°C/350°F/Gas Mark 4. Cook the macaroni in a saucepan of boiling water according to the packet instructions until tender, adding the petits pois and courgette 3 minutes before the end of the cooking time. Drain, reserving the cooking water.

2. Meanwhile, make the cheese sauce. Melt the butter in a small saucepan over a low heat, add the flour and cook for 1 minute. Gradually pour in the milk, stirring continuously until the sauce has thickened. Remove from the heat and stir in the mustard and three-quarters of the cheese. Keep stirring until the cheese has melted.

3. Tip the cooked pasta and vegetables into the sauce, adding 2 tablespoons of the reserved cooking water if necessary, and stir until combined. Spoon into a small ovenproof dish and sprinkle with the remaining cheese. Bake in the oven for 15–20 minutes, or until the cheese has melted.

4. Using the back of a fork, mash the pasta mixture to a coarse purée, adding a little milk if necessary. Alternatively, finely chop.

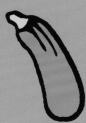
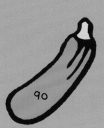

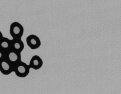

Lovely lamb with mint + pine nuts

serves **4** | prep **15** minutes | cook **35** minutes

Lamb is a great source of iron for growing little brains, and pine nuts are packed with protein. (Oh, and they aren't really nuts at all – they're seeds!)

What you need

75 g/2½ oz **white basmati rice**

75 g/2½ oz **frozen petits pois**

2 teaspoons **olive oil**

125 g/4½ oz lean **minced lamb**

1 small **onion**, finely chopped

1 small **courgette**, diced

1 teaspoon **ground allspice**

20 g/¾ oz **raisins**

3 **tomatoes**, diced

3 tablespoons **pine nuts**, finely chopped

A handful of **mint** leaves, finely chopped

What to do

1. Cook the rice in a saucepan of boiling water according to the packet instructions until tender, adding the peas 3 minutes before the end of the cooking time. Drain and set aside.

2. Meanwhile, heat the oil in a nonstick frying pan over a medium heat and cook the mince for 5 minutes, breaking it up with the back of a fork, until browned all over. Remove with a slotted spoon and set aside.

3. Pour off all but 2 teaspoons of the oil in the pan, add the onion and cook for 5 minutes until softened. Return the lamb to the pan with the courgette, allspice, raisins, tomatoes and 50 ml/2 fl oz boiled water and cover with a lid. Cook for 20 minutes, stirring occasionally, until the lamb is cooked through.

4. Stir in the cooked rice and peas, pine nuts and mint and heat through until piping hot.

5. Using the back of a fork, mash the lamb mixture to a coarse purée, adding a little boiled water if necessary. Alternatively, finely chop.

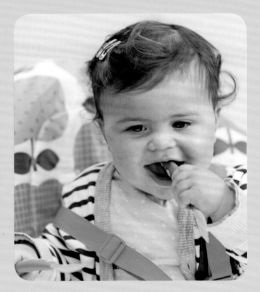

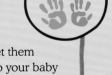 Feed the senses

Pop + squish!

Take out a few cooked peas, let them cool, then hand them whole to your baby to 'pop!' and squish between tiny fingers.

Little explorer's bulgar wheat salad

This super-delicious, baby-friendly salad is perfect for popping in a pot and taking on outdoor adventures with your little explorer.

What you need

25 g/1 oz **bulgar wheat**

½ **courgette**, coarsely grated

5 cm/2 inch piece of **cucumber**, peeled, sliced lengthways, deseeded and diced

3 **tomatoes**

20 g/¾ oz **feta cheese**, grated

2 teaspoons **extra virgin olive oil**

1 teaspoon **lemon juice**

1–2 tablespoons snipped **chives**

What to do

1. Place the bulgar wheat in a saucepan, cover with water and bring to the boil, then reduce the heat, cover with a lid and simmer for 15 minutes, or until very tender. Drain well, then place in a serving bowl.

2. Meanwhile, steam the courgette and cucumber in a saucepan over a medium heat for 5 minutes, adding the tomatoes 2 minutes before the end of the cooking time. Pick out the tomatoes and when cool enough to handle, peel off the skins and finely chop the flesh. Finely chop the courgette and cucumber.

3. Stir the tomatoes, courgette, cucumber, feta, oil, lemon juice and chives into the cooked bulgar. Using the back of a fork, mash the salad to a coarse purée, adding a little boiled water if the texture is too coarse.

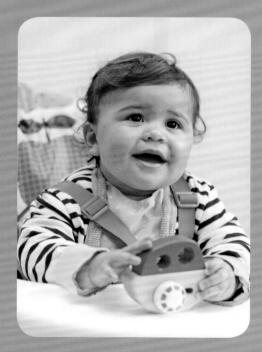

Our friends say...

'I've found that my little girl is more likely to try something if she's been able to squish it or prod it first. Then, it's natural for her to put it in her mouth as part of the learning process.'

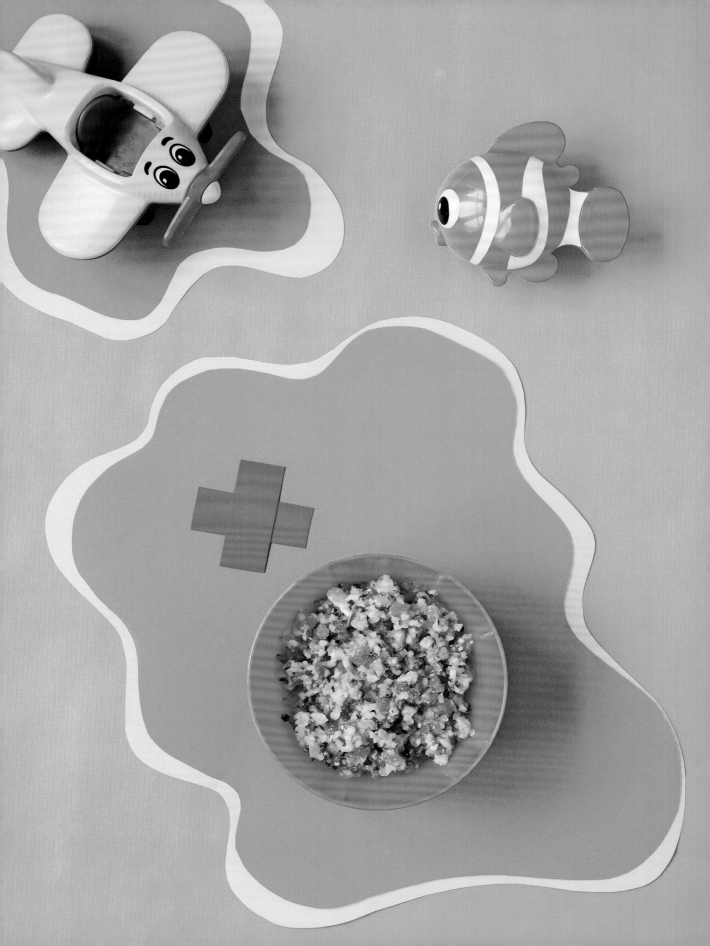

Haddock + pesto pasta bake

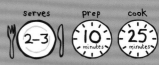

Pasta bake is brilliant for when you have your baby's friends for tea – pop it in the oven and when it's cooked there's enough for everyone. We love it that this one is made using fish, but you could just as easily use bite-sized cooked chicken (or tofu) pieces instead.

What you need

60 g/2¼ oz dried **penne pasta**

2 teaspoons **olive oil**

175 g/6 oz skinless, boneless **haddock fillet**

4 teaspoons **red or green pesto** (see p.54)

6 tablespoons canned **chopped tomatoes**

½ teaspoon **dried oregano**

5 g/⅛ oz **Parmesan cheese**, finely grated

What to do

1. Preheat the oven to 190°C/375°F/Gas Mark 5. Cook the pasta in a saucepan of boiling water according to the packet instructions until tender. Drain, reserving the cooking water.

2. Meanwhile, heat the oil in a small, nonstick frying pan over a medium heat and cook the haddock for 8 minutes, turning once, until cooked through. Remove the fish and flake into large pieces. Remove any bones.

3. Place the pasta, 3 tablespoons of the reserved cooking water, the haddock, pesto, tomatoes and oregano in a bowl and stir gently until combined. Transfer to a small ovenproof dish and sprinkle over the Parmesan. Bake in the oven for 13–15 minutes until the cheese has melted.

4. Using the back of a fork, mash the pasta bake to a coarse purée, adding a little boiled water if necessary. Alternatively, finely chop.

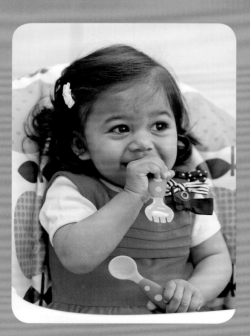

old and new

One good way to offer new flavours, such as new herbs or spices, is to mix them up in foods your baby is already familiar with. And don't forget to offer them lots of times, so that 'new' tastes become familiar, too!

Lemony chicken with sunny Thai noodles

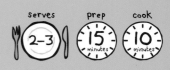

serves 2–3   prep 15 minutes   cook 10 minutes

10+ months

Bring a little ray of sunshine into your kitchen with this simple noodle recipe.
Add in the lemongrass for a fragrant, citrusy flavour that is traditional in Asian cooking.

What you need

40 g/1½ oz **wholewheat noodles**

¼ **red pepper**, cored, deseeded and diced

1 **runner bean**, finely sliced on the diagonal

1 **lemongrass stalk**, peeled and crushed with the blade of a knife

2 teaspoons **sunflower oil**

1 skinless **chicken breast** (about 125 g/4½ oz), cut into thin strips

1 small **garlic** clove, finely chopped

5 tablespoons **coconut milk**

1 tablespoon chopped **basil** leaves

What to do

1. Place the noodles, red pepper, runner bean and lemongrass stalk in a saucepan, cover with plenty of boiling water and cook for 3–5 minutes until tender. Drain, reserving the cooking water, then cool under cold running water. Discard the lemongrass.

2. Meanwhile, heat the oil in a wok or large, nonstick frying pan over a high heat and stir-fry the chicken for 5 minutes until cooked through. Reduce the heat slightly and stir in the garlic, then add the cooked noodles, vegetables, coconut milk and 3 tablespoons of the reserved cooking water to the pan and heat through. Stir in the basil before serving.

3. Using the back of a fork, mash the chicken noodles to a coarse purée, adding a little boiled water if necessary. Alternatively, finely chop.

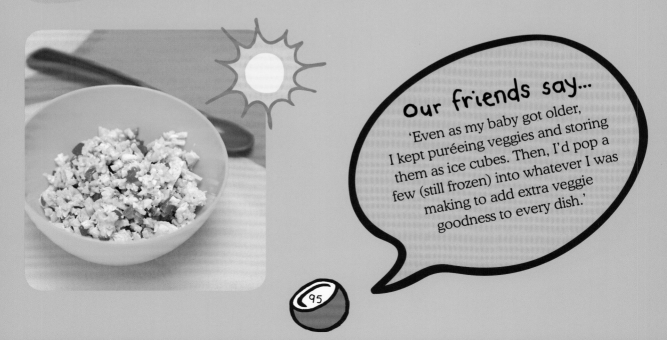

Our friends say...
'Even as my baby got older, I kept puréeing veggies and storing them as ice cubes. Then, I'd pop a few (still frozen) into whatever I was making to add extra veggie goodness to every dish.'

95

Jammin' Jamaican fish curry

serves **4** | prep **20** minutes | cook **25** minutes

Traditional Jamaican flavours infuse this hearty dish and will get little taste buds jammin'. (Why not get out some saucepans and wooden spoons for a jammin' drum session, too?)

What you need

150 g/5½ oz **new potatoes**, scrubbed and halved

2 teaspoons **olive oil**

1 small **onion**, finely chopped

1 small **red pepper**, cored, deseeded and diced

1 large **garlic** clove, chopped

½ teaspoon **ground allspice**

2 teaspoons **mild curry powder**

3 **tomatoes**, deseeded and diced

25 g/1 oz **creamed coconut**, cut into pieces

50 g/1¾ oz **frozen petits pois**

200 g/7 oz thick skinless, boneless **white fish fillet**, such as haddock, bones removed and cut into large bite-sized pieces

White basmati rice, freshly cooked, to serve

What to do

1) Cook the potatoes in a saucepan of boiling water for 12–15 minutes until tender. Drain and leave to dry and cool slightly, then peel off the skins.

2) Meanwhile, heat the oil in a saucepan over a medium–low heat. Add the onion and red pepper, cover with a lid and cook for 10 minutes, stirring occasionally, until softened. Stir in the garlic and add 200 ml/ 7 fl oz water, the spices and tomatoes and bring almost to the boil. Reduce the heat, add the coconut and stir until melted, then part-cover with a lid and simmer for 5 minutes until slightly thickened.

3) Add the petits pois, fish and potatoes and cook gently, uncovered, for a further 5 minutes, or until the fish is cooked through.

4) Using the back of a fork, mash the fish mixture to a coarse purée, adding a little boiled water if necessary. Alternatively, finely chop. Serve with the freshly cooked basmati rice.

Our friends say...

'When a recipe calls for chopping onions, I chop a few extra and put the slices I don't need in the freezer to save time on chopping another day.'

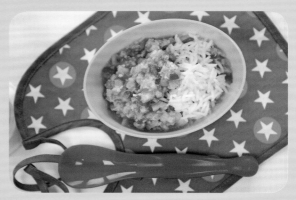

96

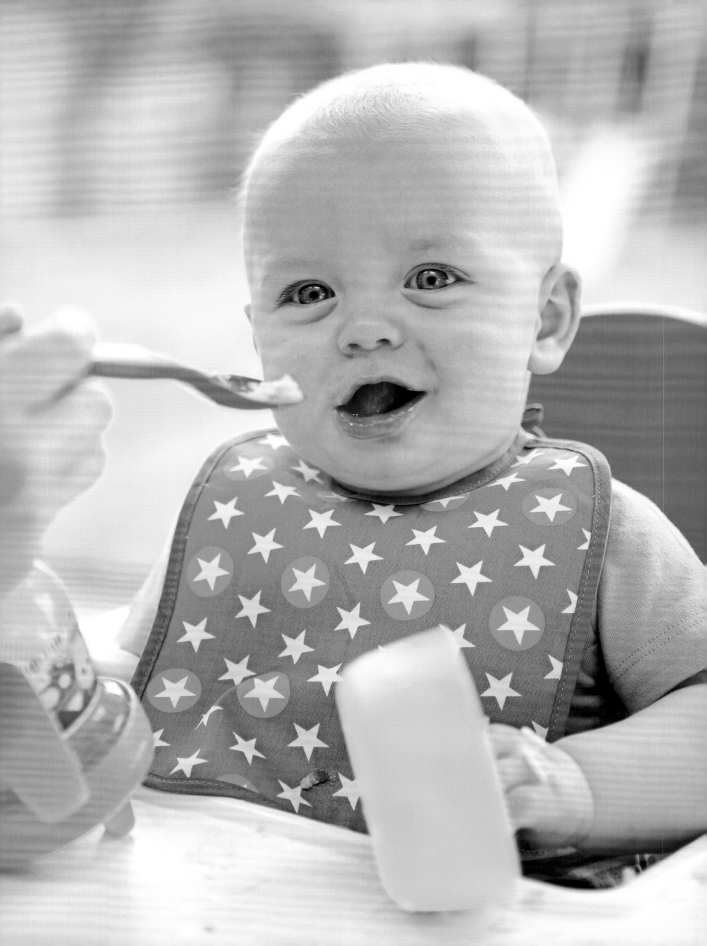

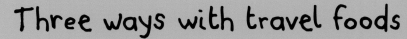

3 ways

Three ways with travel foods

At Ella's Kitchen we love family holidays! Here are some recipes you can make your little one if the only equipment you have is a hotel-room kettle – perfect if you're on an *actual* journey during your weaning journey! All recipes serve one baby aged between 10 and 12 months.

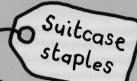

Suitcase staples

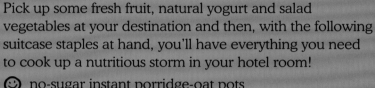

Pick up some fresh fruit, natural yogurt and salad vegetables at your destination and then, with the following suitcase staples at hand, you'll have everything you need to cook up a nutritious storm in your hotel room!

- ☺ no-sugar instant porridge-oat pots
- ☺ couscous
- ☺ dried noodles
- ☺ small cans of tuna, salmon or pulses
- ☺ dried fruit (such as jumbo raisins) and canned fruit

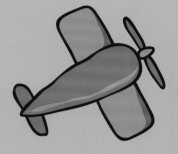

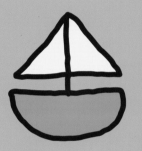

Fruity funtime porridge

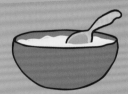

What you need

70 g/2½ oz pot no-sugar **instant oats**

225 g/8 oz can **chopped fruit in juice** (such as peaches, apricots or clementines), drained

A handful of **jumbo raisins**

1 tablespoon **natural yogurt**, to serve (optional)

What to do

1. Pour boiling water over the oats (straight into the instant pot is usually fine, but check first). Leave to stand for 2 minutes, or according to the packet instructions.

2. Add the canned fruit and the raisins and stir well to combine. Allow to cool slightly, then serve topped with a spoonful of yogurt, if using.

Seaside salmon + avocado couscous

What you need

4 tablespoons **couscous**

105 g/3½ oz can **red salmon**

3 cm/1¼ in piece **cucumber**, finely diced

½ **avocado**, mashed

What to do

1. Place the couscous in a bowl and add 4 tablespoons of just-boiled water. Cover with a plate for 10 minutes, then remove the plate and fluff up the grains with a fork.

2. Add the salmon, cucumber and mashed avocado to the couscous, mix well to combine and serve immediately.

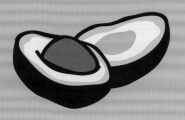

Wriggly noodles, sweetcorn + sardines

What you need

1 nest of dried **fine egg noodles**

95 g/3¼ oz can **sardines in tomato sauce**

4 tablespoons drained no-salt, no-sugar canned **sweetcorn**

What to do

1. Place the noodles in a bowl, cover with just-boiled water and leave to soak for 5–6 minutes, until soft. Meanwhile, mash the sardines in their sauce.

2. Drain off the excess water from the noodles, then add the sardines and the sweetcorn and mix well until the noodles are coated with the tomato sauce and everything is combined. Serve immediately.

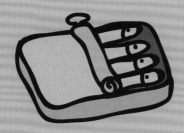

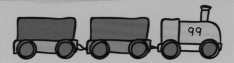

Mushroom, pea + tomato pilaf

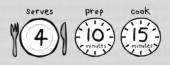

Some say that pilaf is rice at its very, very best – fluffy, and lightly flavoured with turmeric and coriander to make it very, very yummy.

What you need

75 g/2½ oz **white basmati rice**

75 g/2½ oz **frozen petits pois**

2 teaspoons **olive oil**

1 small **onion**, finely chopped

55 g/2 oz **mushrooms**, chopped

2 **tomatoes**, deseeded and diced

1 teaspoon **turmeric**

1 teaspoon **ground coriander**

2 tablespoons chopped **flat-leaf parsley** (optional)

2 hard-boiled **eggs**, halved

What to do

1) Cook the rice in a saucepan of boiling water according to the packet instructions until tender, adding the petits pois 3 minutes before the end of the cooking time. Drain.

2) Meanwhile, heat the oil in a nonstick frying pan over a medium heat and cook the onion for 5 minutes, stirring frequently, until softened. Add the mushrooms and tomatoes and cook for a further 5 minutes until tender.

3) Add the turmeric and coriander, then the cooked rice and peas, and the parsley (if using). Top each portion with half a hard-boiled egg.

4) Using the back of a fork, mash the pilaf to a coarse purée, adding a little boiled water if necessary. Alternatively, finely chop.

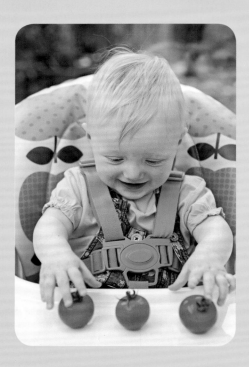

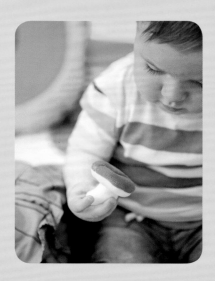

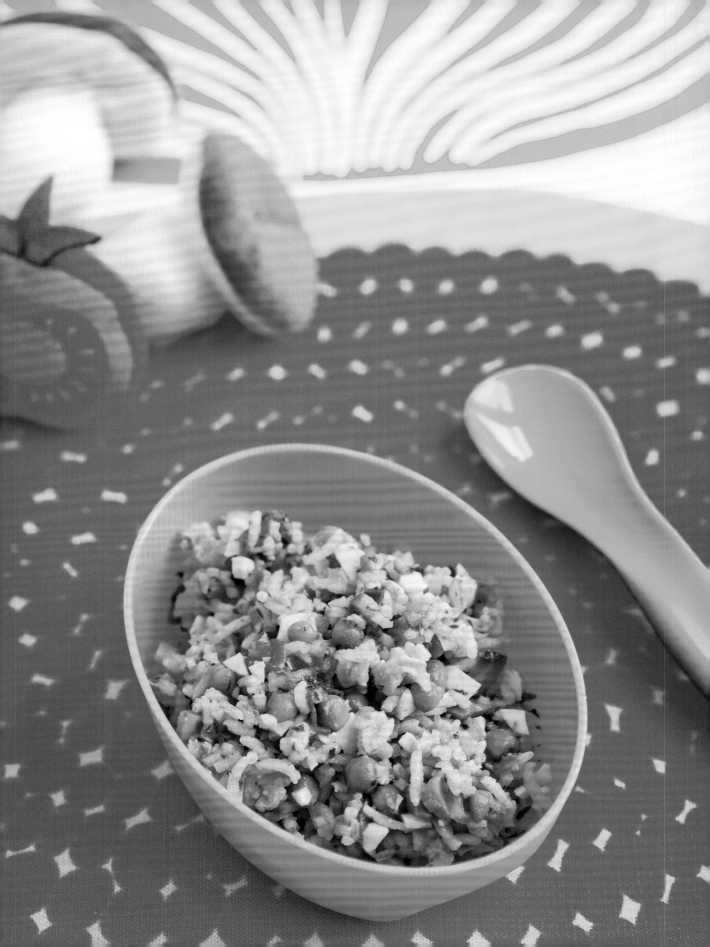

Golden shepherd's pie

serves **4** | prep **20** minutes | cook **55** minutes

We've spiced up this mealtime favourite by adding cumin and ginger...
and we've given it a boost of green veggies, too.

What you need

2 teaspoons **olive oil**

125 g/4½ oz lean **minced lamb**

1 small **onion**, finely chopped

1 **carrot**, peeled and grated

75 g/2½ oz **spring cabbage**,
finely chopped

2 **garlic** cloves, chopped

½ teaspoon **ground cumin**

1 teaspoon **ground ginger**

2 teaspoons **balsamic vinegar**

1 tablespoon **tomato purée**

250 g/9 oz **sweet potatoes**,
peeled and cubed

2 tablespoons **whole milk**

10 g/¼ oz **unsalted butter**,
cut into small pieces

What to do

1. Preheat the oven to 180°C/350°F/Gas Mark 4. Heat the oil in a saucepan over a medium heat and cook the lamb for 5 minutes, breaking it up with the back of a fork, until browned all over. Remove the lamb using a slotted spoon and set aside.

2. Pour off all but 2 teaspoons of the oil in the pan and cook the onion, carrot and cabbage for 8 minutes, stirring frequently, until softened. Reduce the heat slightly and stir in the garlic, then return the lamb to the pan with the cumin, ginger, vinegar, tomato purée and 150 ml/¼ pint boiled water and stir well. Cover with a lid and cook for 15 minutes until cooked through.

3. Meanwhile, cook the sweet potatoes in a saucepan of boiling water for 10–15 minutes until tender, then drain and return to the pan. Add the milk and mash until smooth.

4. Spoon the lamb mixture into a small ovenproof dish and top with the mash. Dot the butter on top and bake in the oven for 25 minutes until starting to crisp on top.

5. Using the back of the fork, mash the shepherd's pie to a coarse purée, adding a little boiled water if necessary. Alternatively, finely chop.

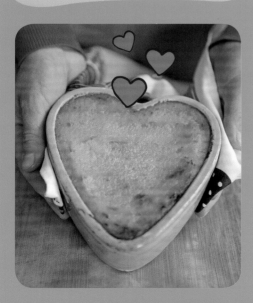

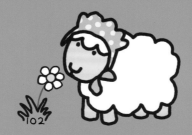

Groovy greens + beef noodles

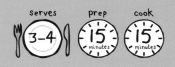

serves 3–4 · prep 15 minutes · cook 15 minutes

This is Ella's Kitchen's very own take on a classic Chinese beef chow mein. Just as you'd expect, it's packed with colourful veggies and tantalizing tastes to tickle little taste buds.

What you need

60 g/2¼ oz dried **egg noodles**

3 small **broccoli** florets

2 teaspoons **sunflower oil**

125 g/4½ oz lean **beef strips**

1 **garlic** clove, chopped

1 cm/½ inch piece of **root ginger**, peeled and very finely chopped

1 large **spring onion**, finely chopped

¼ **red pepper**, cored, deseeded and finely chopped

40 g/1½ oz **spring cabbage**, finely chopped

50 ml/2 fl oz **fresh apple juice**

½ teaspoon reduced-salt **soy sauce**

What to do

1. Cook the noodles and broccoli in a saucepan of boiling water for 3–5 minutes until tender. Drain, reserving the cooking water. Cool the noodles and broccoli under running water.

2. Heat the oil in a wok or small, nonstick frying pan over a high heat and stir-fry the beef for 3 minutes until browned all over. Add the garlic, ginger, spring onion, red pepper and cabbage and stir-fry for a further 3 minutes until softened.

3. Pour in the apple juice, 50 ml/2 fl oz of the reserved cooking water and the soy sauce. Add the cooked noodles and broccoli and heat through for 2 minutes.

4. Using the back of a fork, mash the noodle mixture to a coarse purée, adding more of the reserved cooking water if necessary. Alternatively, finely chop.

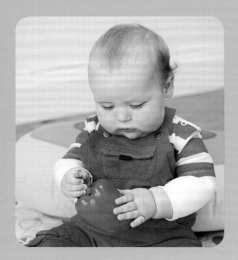

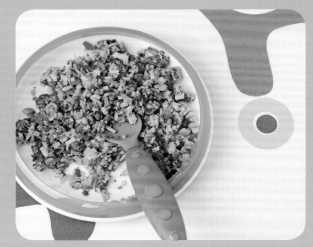

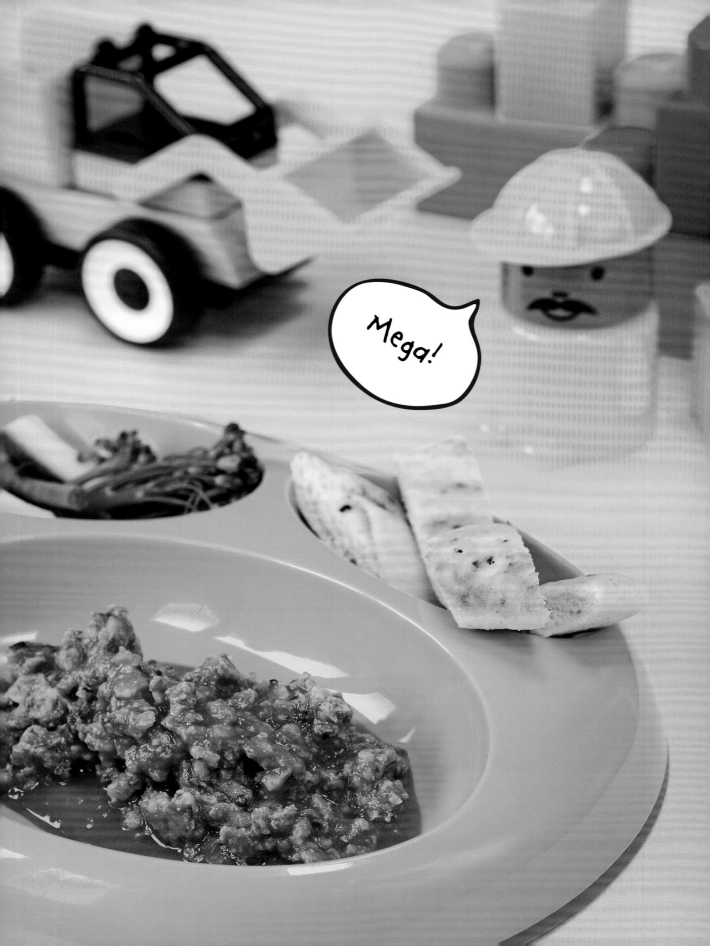

Mega meatballs with mango sauce

Meatballs as you've never seen them before! The mango sauce gives them a delicious tang and they're just the perfect size for little hands to grab and hold. You could also try serving them with minty yogurt dip (see p.180).

What you need

75 g/2½ oz lean **minced beef**

1 teaspoon **mild curry powder**

1 tablespoon finely chopped **coriander** (optional)

20 g/¾ oz **fresh breadcrumbs**

1 small **egg**, lightly beaten

Olive oil, for frying

Green vegetables and **naan bread**, cut into fingers, to serve

For the mango sauce

1 small **garlic** clove, chopped

5 mm/¼ inch piece of **root ginger**, peeled and very finely chopped

2 teaspoons **olive oil**

300 g/10½ oz canned **chopped tomatoes**

80 g/2¾ oz peeled and stoned **mango**, cut into small pieces

What to do

1. Place the mince, curry powder, coriander (if using) and breadcrumbs in a bowl and stir until combined. Add enough of the beaten egg to bind everything together (you won't need it all). Divide the mixture into 6 walnut-sized pieces and shape into meatballs. Transfer to a plate, cover with clingfilm and chill for 20 minutes to firm up slightly.

2. Meanwhile, make the sauce. Heat the garlic and ginger in the oil in a saucepan over a medium–low heat for 1 minute. Add the tomatoes, part-cover with a lid and simmer for 10 minutes until reduced and thickened. Stir in the mango and heat through. Purée the sauce in a food processor, or using a hand blender, until smooth. Set aside.

3. Heat enough oil to coat the base of a large, nonstick frying pan and cook the meatballs in 2 batches each for 10 minutes, turning occasionally, until browned all over and cooked through.

4. Warm the mango sauce if necessary, then serve with the meatballs. Using the back of a fork, mash the meatballs and sauce to a coarse purée, adding a little boiled water if necessary. Alternatively, finely chop. Serve with vegetables and fingers of naan bread.

Ella's shortcut

For a super-speedy mango sauce use a 70 g/2 oz pouch of Ella's Kitchen mangoes, mangoes, mangoes instead!

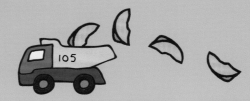

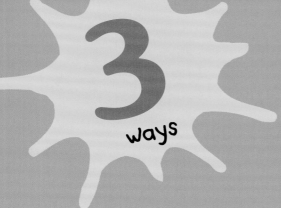

Three ways with baked + scooped potatoes

Baked potatoes make such an easy and nutritious teatime favourite. Our clever fillings are simple to put together, then all mashed in with the creamy potato flesh and served in a bowl. Little ones can't manage the potato skins until after 12 months – so, nibble them as your own tasty snack at baby's teatime instead!

Baby's baked potatoes

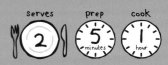

serves 2 · prep 5 minutes · cook 1 hour

2 small **potatoes** (about 115 g/4 oz each), scrubbed

Filling (see below) and **favourite vegetables**, to serve

1. Preheat the oven to 200°C/400°F/Gas Mark 6. Place a skewer through each potato to speed up the cooking time, then bake in the oven for about 1 hour or until cooked through.

2. When the potatoes are ready, cut each one in half, then scoop the flesh into a bowl. Add your chosen filling and mash together. Serve with favourite veg.

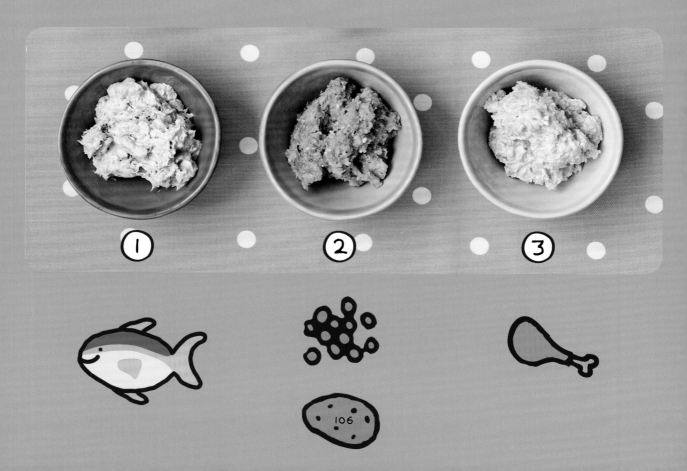

① ② ③

106

① Tuna, cheese + chive filling

serves 2 | **prep** 5 minutes | **cook** no cook

3 tablespoons drained canned **tuna chunks** in spring water

1 tablespoon **cream cheese**

2 tablespoons **natural yogurt**

1 tablespoon snipped **chives**

① Mash the tuna in a bowl and mix in the cream cheese, yogurt and chives.

② Pea pesto filling

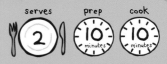

serves 2 | **prep** 5 minutes | **cook** 5 minutes

100 g/3½ oz **frozen peas**

2 teaspoons **red or green pesto** (see p.54)

1 teaspoon **olive oil**

10 g/¼ oz **Cheddar cheese**, finely grated

① Steam or boil the peas in a saucepan over a medium heat for 3 minutes until tender.

② Purée the peas with the pesto, oil, cheese and 1 tablespoon of boiled water in a food processor, or using a hand blender, until smooth. To make the purée smoother, pass it through a sieve after blending.

③ Chicken + vegetable filling

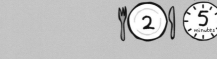

serves 2 | **prep** 10 minutes | **cook** 10 minutes

1 **carrot**, peeled and thinly sliced

3 tablespoons no-salt, no-sugar canned **sweetcorn**, drained

3 tablespoons **natural yogurt**

25 g/1 oz **cooked chicken**, finely chopped

① Steam or boil the carrot in a saucepan over a medium heat for 8 minutes until tender.

② Roughly chop the carrot, then transfer to a food processor or blender.

③ Add the sweetcorn, yogurt and chicken with 1 tablespoon of boiled water and whiz to a coarse purée.

Stacked + packed veggie moussaka

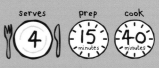

serves 4 | prep 15 minutes | cook 40 minutes

This is a classic Greek recipe that bursts with 5 different veggies as well as a super-pulse. Wow, that really is stacked and packed!

What you need

- 1 small **aubergine**, peeled and cut into bite-sized chunks
- 1 tablespoon **olive oil**
- 1 small **onion**, finely chopped
- ½ **red pepper**, cored, deseeded and diced
- 2 **garlic** cloves, chopped
- 2 teaspoons **dried oregano**
- 400 g/14 oz can **chopped tomatoes**
- 2 **sun-dried tomatoes** in oil, drained and very finely chopped
- 100 g/3½ oz **canned green lentils** in water, drained
- 55 g/2 oz **mozzarella cheese**, torn into small pieces

What to do

1. Preheat the oven to 190°C/375°/Gas Mark 5. Steam the aubergine in a saucepan over a medium heat for 8 minutes, or until tender.

2. Meanwhile, heat the oil in a saucepan over a medium–low heat. Add the onion and red pepper, cover with a lid and cook for 10 minutes, stirring occasionally, until softened. Add the garlic, cooked aubergine and oregano and cook for a further 2 minutes.

3. Add the chopped tomatoes, sun-dried tomatoes and lentils, part-cover with the lid and simmer, stirring occasionally, for 10 minutes until the sauce has reduced and thickened.

4. Spoon the tomato sauce into a small ovenproof dish and scatter the mozzarella over. Bake in the oven for 15–18 minutes until the mozzarella has melted.

5. Using the back of a fork, mash the moussaka to a coarse purée, adding a little boiled water if necessary. Alternatively, finely chop.

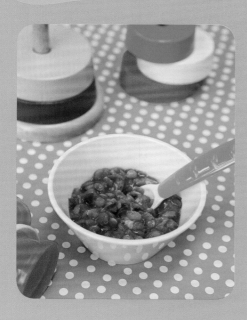

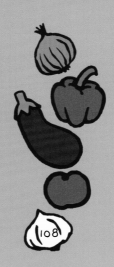

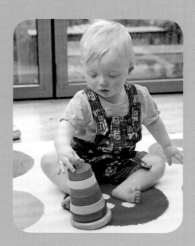

Chilly cherry pudding pots

serves **4** · prep **15** minutes · cook **10** minutes + standing

Our treat-time cherry pots are great for introducing your baby to warming spices. Cherries are packed with vitamin C for healthy immunity.

What you need

200 g/7 oz **frozen stoned dark cherries**

2 tablespoons **fresh apple juice**

1 teaspoon **ground mixed spice**

4 slices day-old **half-white and half-wholemeal bread**

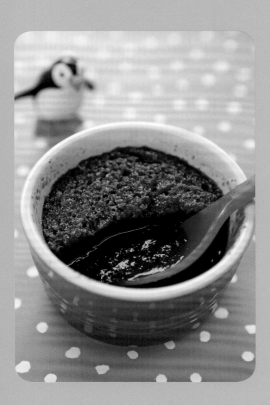

What to do

1. Put the cherries in a saucepan with the apple juice, mixed spice and 2 tablespoons of water. Cover and cook over a medium–low heat for 5–7 minutes until the cherries are soft.

2. Meanwhile, using a 7 cm/2¾ inch ramekin as a cutter, stamp out 2 rounds in each slice of bread. Place a round in the bottom of each ramekin and set aside.

3. Strain the cherries, reserving the juice in a jug. Purée the cherries in a food processor or using a hand blender until smooth.

4. Spoon 1 tablespoon of the juice evenly over the bread in each ramekin, pressing it into the bread. Top with the puréed cherries and then another round of bread. Spoon over the remaining juice and gently press down. If you can, leave the puddings for 30 minutes to let the flavours mingle before serving. The pots will keep in the fridge for up to 3 days.

Crumb-tastic

Pop any leftover bread in a food processor and whiz it up into breadcrumbs. You can store the breadcrumbs in a container in the freezer until you need them – try them in our Jumping Bean Burgers on page 118.

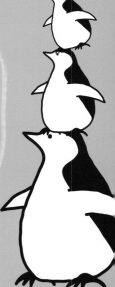

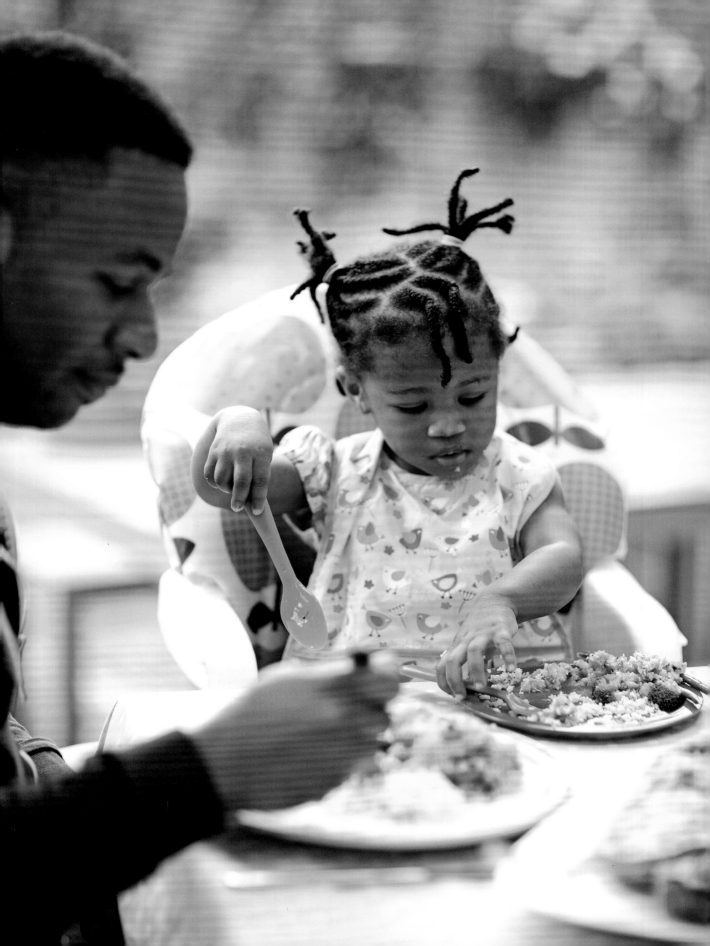

Mega meals for one + all

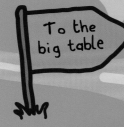
To the big table

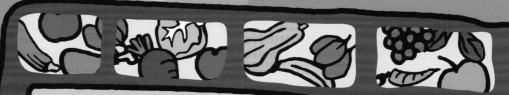

You've made it to the big table! From 12 months old, you can start eating grown-up meals and sharing your foody adventures with all your family.

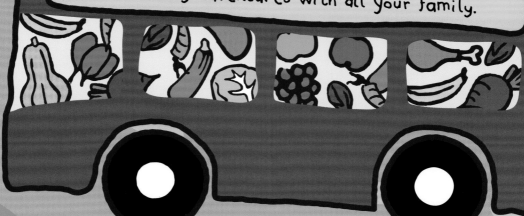

12 months + beyond

By the time babies reach their first birthday, they are increasingly independent little people and will especially love having a spoon – and lots of encouragement – so that they can feed themselves. Many recipes in this chapter are intended for you to enjoy as a family – your baby learns from you, so try to eat together as often as you can.

What to give

At around a year, growth rates slow down, but babies tend to be much more active. The two more or less balance each other out and your baby's appetite probably won't grow too much. Even so, keep healthy snacks on hand to keep your busy baby going between meals. (Hungry babies can get very cross!)

At around 12 months little ones can start to become fussy about what they eat. This means that they may start to reject foods they previously liked, or refuse to try new foods. Red meats and green veggies are often the first casualties, but that means your little one might not be getting enough iron and B-vitamins. Wholegrain cereals, such as oats, and wholegrain bread are great sources of B-vitamins, while also providing fibre (which is important for keeping little digestive systems healthy). There are B-vitamins in eggs, too – try them scrambled or made into omelettes or frittatas for protein-rich finger-food meals. Dried fruits, such as dried apricots and raisins, are rich in iron, while also allowing little ones to practise their pincer grip.

(Don't feel you need to offer fibre at every meal – too much fibre can fill up babies too quickly, squashing their appetites for the other nutrients they need.)

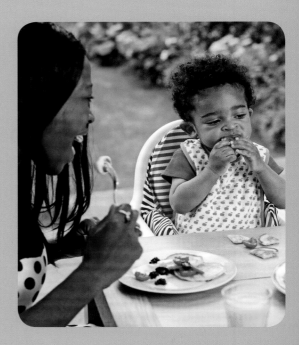

Milky newsflash!

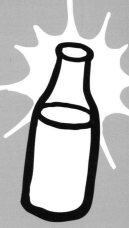

From 12 months old, your little one can have whole (full-fat) cow's milk as a drink, all on its own – delicious calcium-rich goodness for strong bones and teeth, in a cup. Perfect!

Tips on texture

By a year old most babies have many of their first 'cutting' teeth (the incisors, at the front). This means they're ready for plates of food that are chopped-up versions of the foods you would eat – and there's no need to mix these with purées any more. Molars come through usually between 12 and 18 months – these are the chewing teeth, and once your baby has them, you can introduce foods with a harder texture. Yipp*eee*!

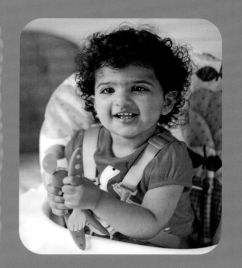

How much?

During their first year, little ones grow at an immense rate. Now that rate is slowing down and most will eat roughly the same amount at mealtimes as they were eating at 10 months (see p.81) – but may need regular snacks. It's still most important to allow your baby's appetite to guide you. Older babies are more ready than ever to listen to their bodies and stop when they feel full. Listening now makes them less likely to overeat when they're older.

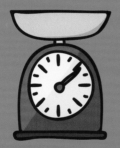

Tingling taste buds

Your baby is now ready to eat almost anything, as long as it's chopped up. If your little one shows an interest – have a go! (Of course, naughty whole nuts are still off the menu.) At 1 year old, your baby can also now enjoy the sweetness of honey as a little treat – our Stripy Berry Puds (see p.149) are a delicious way to start!

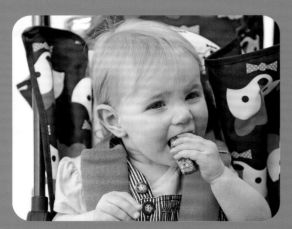

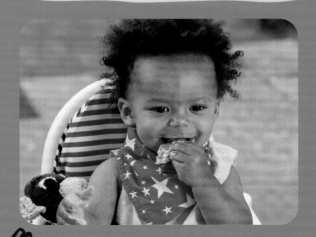

Wakey-wakey cranberry muesli

makes **20** portions · prep **15** minutes · cook **10** minutes

Nothing beats homemade muesli and this one is packed full of sunny sunflower seeds and buttery pecans for a truly delicious start to the day.

What you need

- 100 g/3½ oz **pecan nut** halves
- 200 g/7 oz **porridge oats**
- 3 tablespoons **sunflower seeds**
- 100 g/3½ oz small **dried fruit**, such as **raisins**, **sultanas** or **cranberries**, chopped as necessary
- 1 tablespoon **sesame seeds**
- **Baby's usual milk**, to serve

What to do

1. Dry-fry the pecans in a large, nonstick frying pan over a medium–low heat for 3–4 minutes, turning occasionally, until toasted (don't let them burn). Tip into a bowl and leave to cool.

2. Put the oats in the pan and dry-fry over a medium–low heat for 4–5 minutes, stirring frequently, until slightly browned. Leave to cool.

3. Whiz the pecans and sunflower seeds in a food processor or blender until finely chopped, then transfer to a bowl. Place the oats in the processor and coarsely chop. Add to the bowl with the remaining dry ingredients and mix together. Store in an airtight container. Serve with milk (leave to soften in the milk for a few minutes before serving, if necessary).

Just-for-me creamy eggs

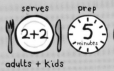

serves **2+2** adults + kids · prep **5** minutes · cook **15** minutes

These little baked egg pots are really simple to prepare. They make an exciting (and creamy) alternative to boiled eggs.

What you need

- 4 **eggs**
- 4 teaspoons **crème fraîche**
- 20 g/¾ oz **Cheddar cheese**, grated
- **Bread**, toasted, to serve

What to do

1. Preheat the oven to 180°C/350°F/Gas Mark 4. Crack each egg into a separate ramekin and top with 1 teaspoon of the crème fraîche and a sprinkling of cheese.

2. Place the ramekins in a baking tray and bake in the oven for 15 minutes, or until set. Serve with fingers of toast.

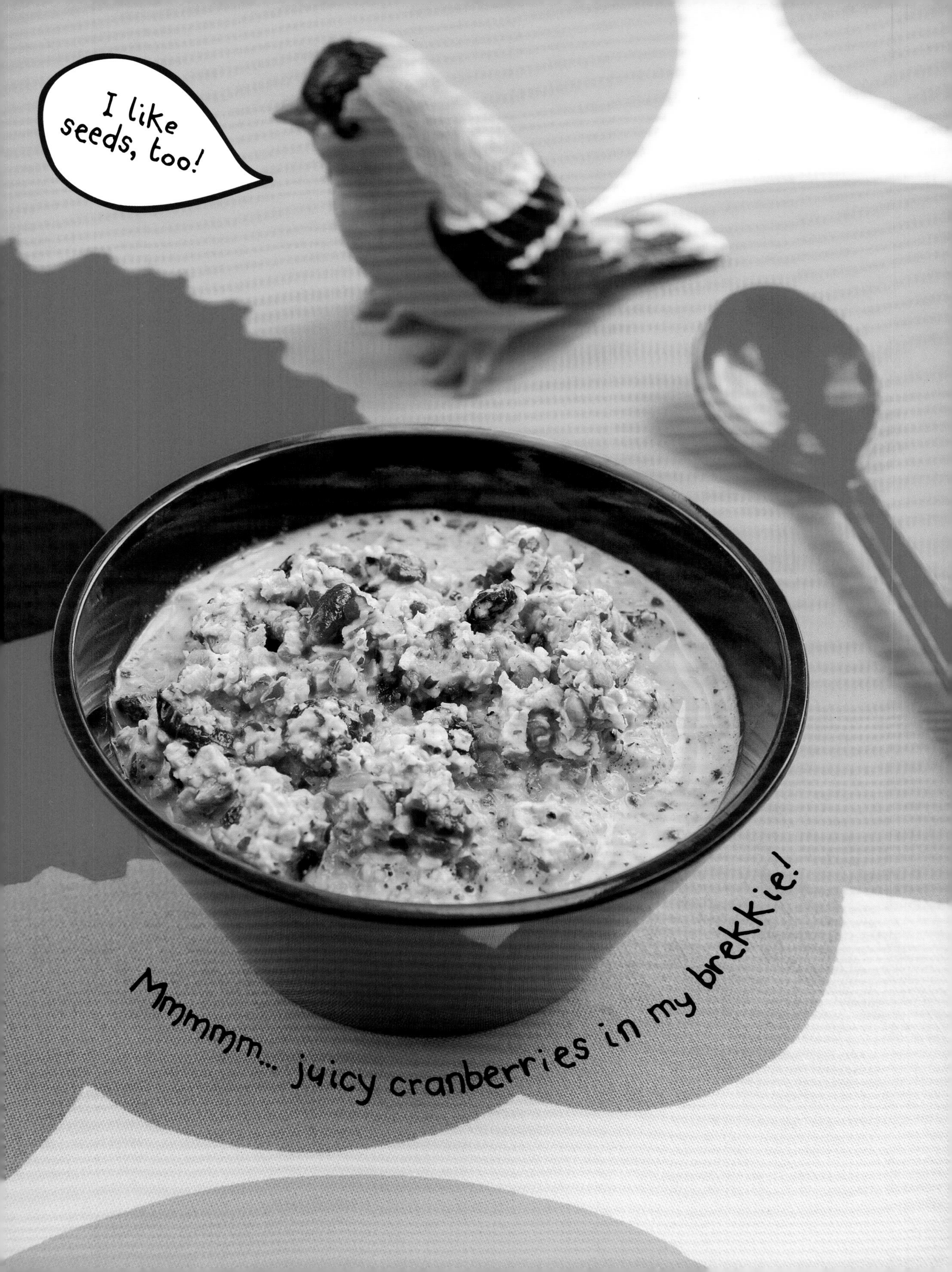
I like seeds, too!
Mmmmm... juicy cranberries in my brekkie!

Chunky monkey pancakes

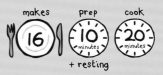

makes 16 | prep 10 minutes + resting | cook 20 minutes

These fluffy pancakes are just right for little fingers to hold. Cottage cheese and banana give them protein and fibre, making them the perfect start for your cheeky monkey.

What you need

170 g/6 oz **plain flour**

1½ teaspoons **baking powder**

1 large **egg**

175 ml/6 fl oz **whole milk**

15 g/½ oz **unsalted butter**, melted, plus extra for cooking

3 tablespoons **cottage cheese**

1 small ripe **banana**, mashed

Fruit and **natural yogurt**, to serve

What to do

1. Sift the flour and baking powder into a large bowl and make a well in the centre.

2. Whisk together the egg and milk in a jug, then stir in the melted butter and cottage cheese. Gradually pour the egg mixture into the flour, whisking continuously to make a smooth batter. Leave to rest for 15 minutes, then stir in the banana.

3. Melt a knob of butter in a large, nonstick frying pan over a medium heat. Add 2 tablespoons of the batter mix per pancake (you should be able to cook 4 at a time). Cook the pancakes for about 2 minutes on each side, reducing the heat slightly if they begin to brown too quickly and adding more butter when needed. Remove from the pan and keep warm in a low oven. Repeat with the remaining ingredients.

4. Serve the pancakes, cut into quarters for babies, with fruit and yogurt.

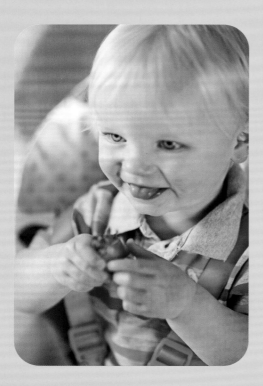

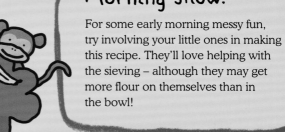

Can I help?

Morning snow!

For some early morning messy fun, try involving your little ones in making this recipe. They'll love helping with the sieving – although they may get more flour on themselves than in the bowl!

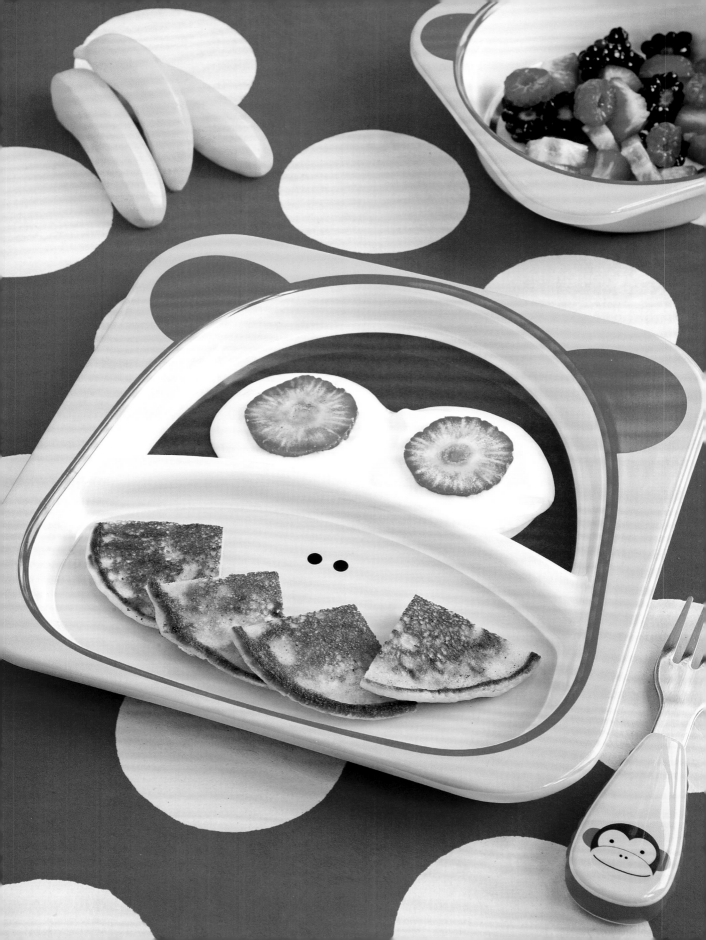

Jumping bean burgers

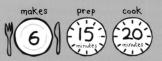

Little taste buds will jump for joy when they get their first try of Mexican spice. You can cook these mini veggie burgers straight from frozen (just increase the cooking time accordingly), so pop any extras in the freezer for another day.

What you need

1½ tablespoons **olive oil**

1 small **onion**, finely chopped

1 large **garlic** clove, finely chopped

400 g/14 oz can **red kidney beans** in water, drained

50 g/1¾ oz **fresh breadcrumbs**

1 heaped teaspoon no-salt **Mexican spice blend**

2 tablespoons **tomato purée**

2 tablespoons **plain flour**, plus extra for dusting

Small warmed **pitta breads**, split open, sliced **tomato** and finely grated **carrot**, to serve

What to do

1. Heat 2 teaspoons of the oil in a large, nonstick frying pan over a medium heat and cook the onion for 8 minutes, stirring frequently, until softened. Add the garlic and cook for a further 1 minute.

2. Meanwhile, using the back of a fork, mash the beans in a large bowl until almost smooth, then stir in the cooked onion and garlic, and the breadcrumbs, Mexican spice blend and tomato purée and stir well until combined.

3. Place the flour in a shallow bowl and dust your hands with a little extra flour. Divide the bean mixture into 6 equal pieces and shape them into burgers. Lightly dust each burger in the flour until coated all over.

4. Heat the remaining oil in the frying pan over a medium heat and cook the burgers for 3 minutes on each side until golden and warmed through. Serve each in a warmed pitta bread with slices of tomato and grated carrot. Finely chop the burgers and tomatoes for babies, if necessary.

Our friends say...

'I make my breadcrumbs in batches and then freeze them, ready for when I need them. They're great not only for making homemade burgers, but for fishcakes and breaded chicken strips, too.'

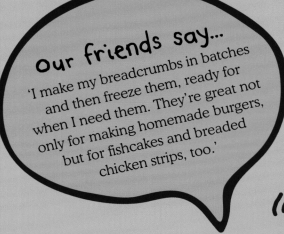

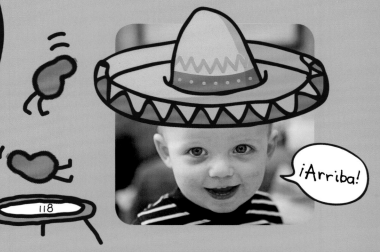

¡Arriba!

Really special rice + prawns

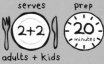

What makes this dish really special? Brown rice is high in fibre and prawns are high in selenium, a mighty mineral that helps build immune systems.

What you need

200 g/7 oz **brown rice**

140 g/5 oz **broccoli**, cut into small florets

1 tablespoon **sunflower oil**

1 onion, **chopped**

1 small **red pepper**, cored, deseeded and diced

2 cm/¾ inch piece of fresh **root ginger**, peeled and very finely chopped

2 **garlic** cloves, finely chopped

2 teaspoons **Chinese 5-spice**

100 g/3½ oz **frozen petits pois**

1 teaspoon reduced-salt **soy sauce**

2 **eggs**, lightly beaten

A handful of **coriander** leaves, chopped

2 teaspoons **sesame oil**

225 g/8 oz **raw peeled prawns**, defrosted if frozen, cut into thirds

What to do

1. Place the rice in a saucepan, cover with 400 ml/14 fl oz water and bring to the boil. Reduce the heat to its lowest setting, cover with a lid and simmer for 20–25 minutes until the rice is tender and the water is absorbed.

2. Meanwhile, steam or boil the broccoli in a saucepan over a medium heat for 5 minutes until tender. Cool under cold running water, drain and set aside.

3. Heat the sunflower oil in a wok or large, nonstick frying pan over a medium–high heat and stir-fry the onion for 3 minutes until softened. Add the red pepper, ginger, garlic, 5-spice and petits pois and stir-fry for 3 minutes until cooked through. Stir in the rice and broccoli and heat thoroughly for 2 minutes, stirring continuously. Stir in the soy sauce.

4. Make a well in the centre of the rice, add the eggs and, when the egg starts to cook, gradually fold it into the rice mixture for 3 minutes until cooked. Stir in the coriander, cover with a lid and leave to stand.

5. Meanwhile, heat the sesame oil in a separate nonstick frying pan and stir-fry the prawns for 3 minutes until pink and cooked through. Stir the prawns into the rice and serve.

Our friends say...

'My baby loves playing colour snap with food. "Snap!" for red peppers and red strawberries, and green peas and green broccoli... and anything else that matches!'

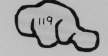

119

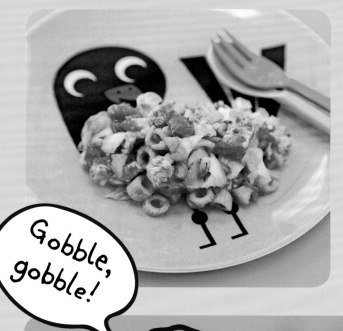

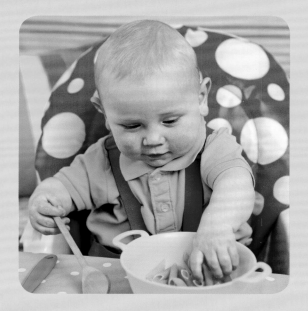

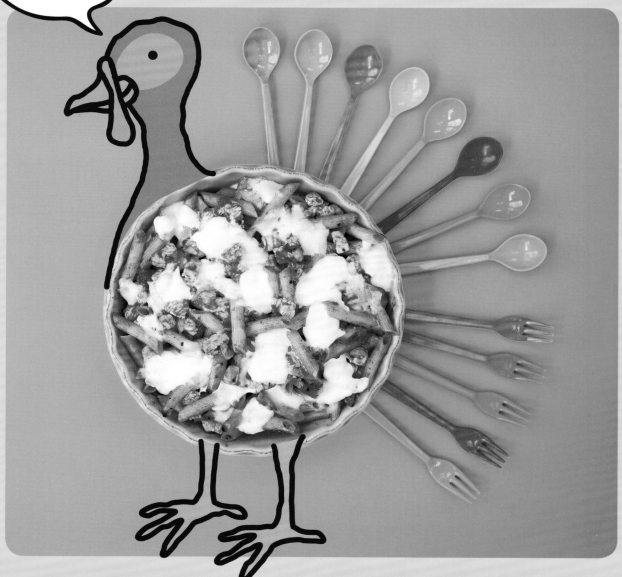

Tuck-in turkey + fennel pasta bake

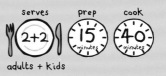

This pasta bake is great for the whole family and introduces your little one to the distinctive taste of fennel. It's also fun to see who can make their mozzarella stre*eeetch* the furthest!

What you need

1 tablespoon **olive oil**

400 g/14 oz skinless **turkey breast**, cut into bite-sized pieces

2 **garlic** cloves, finely chopped

2 teaspoons **dried oregano**

½ teaspoon **fennel seeds**

400 g/14 oz can **chopped tomatoes**

1 tablespoon **tomato purée**

280 g/10 oz dried **penne pasta**

125 g/4½ oz **mozzarella cheese**, torn into pieces

What to do

1. Preheat the oven to 190°C/375°F/Gas Mark 5. Heat the oil in a nonstick frying pan over a medium–high heat and cook the turkey for 5 minutes, turning occasionally, until browned. Remove with a slotted spoon and set aside.

2. Reduce the heat to medium–low, add the garlic, oregano and fennel seeds to the pan and stir, then add the tomatoes and tomato purée. Bring to the boil, then reduce the heat, part-cover with a lid and simmer for 10 minutes, stirring frequently, until reduced and thickened.

3. Meanwhile, cook the pasta in a saucepan of boiling water for about 1 minute less than the packet instructions, or until just tender. Drain, reserving the cooking water.

4. Return the pasta and 4 tablespoons of the reserved cooking water to the saucepan, stir in the turkey and the tomato sauce and warm through. Tip the pasta mixture into an ovenproof dish and scatter the mozzarella over the top.

5. Cover with a lid or aluminium foil and bake for 10 minutes, then remove the lid or foil and cook for a further 10 minutes until the mozzarella has melted and the turkey is cooked through. Finely chop the pasta bake for babies before serving.

Just for fun

Handy turkey

Make a turkey picture! Draw around your little one's hand on a piece of card – the thumb makes the neck and the fingers the plumes. Add a beak, a wattle, a wing and some legs, then help your little one colour it in. Finish it off with a googly eye.

Pizza-tata

serves
2+2
adults + kids
prep
15
minutes
cook
30
minutes

What do you get if you cross a pizza and a frittata? This super-tasty pizza-tata, of course! Get little noses twitching with a sniff of fresh basil.

What you need

150 g/5½ oz **potatoes**, peeled and quartered

1 tablespoon **olive oil**

1 large **onion**, diced

2 **garlic** cloves, finely chopped

1 teaspoon **dried oregano**

7 **eggs**, lightly beaten

85 g/3 oz **mozzarella cheese**, torn into pieces

4 teaspoons **red or green pesto** (see p.54)

5 **cherry tomatoes**, halved

A handful of **pitted black olives** (not in brine), quartered

A few torn **basil** leaves (optional)

Steamed **vegetables**, to serve

What to do

1. Steam or boil the potato in a saucepan over a medium heat for 12–15 minutes until tender. Drain, if necessary, and leave to cool slightly, then cut into small chunks.

2. Meanwhile, heat the oil in a nonstick, ovenproof frying pan over a medium heat. Cook the onion for 8 minutes, stirring frequently, until softened. Stir in the garlic and oregano and cook for a further 1 minute.

3. Meanwhile, preheat the grill to medium–high. Pour the eggs into the pan, add the potato, pressing it down into the egg mixture, and cook over a medium–low heat for 8 minutes, or until the base is set and light golden.

4. Scatter over the mozzarella and dot with the pesto. Top with the tomatoes, olives and basil (if using) and grill for 3–4 minutes until the cheese has melted and the egg is cooked. Leave to stand for a couple of minutes before cutting into wedges, or fingers for babies. Serve with steamed favourite veggies.

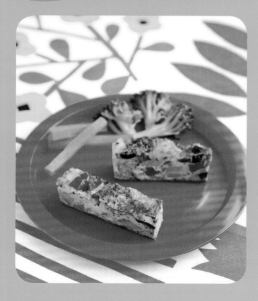
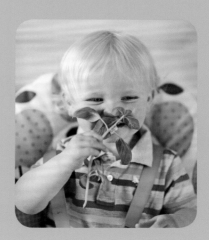

Big smiles cheesy pie

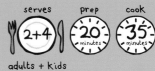

serves 2+4 adults + kids | prep 20 minutes | cook 35 minutes

The best pies are filled to bursting and this one is no exception. It has 5 different types of veg all under one potato roof – it's bound to bring on big smiles all round!

What you need

1 tablespoon **olive oil**

60 g/2¼ oz **swede** or **parsnip**, peeled and diced

2 **carrots**, peeled and diced

1 large **leek**, trimmed, cleaned and sliced

2 large **garlic** cloves, chopped

400 g/14 oz can **chopped tomatoes**

400 g/14 oz can **green lentils** in water, drained

1 teaspoon **dried mixed herbs**

550 g/1 lb 4 oz **potatoes**, peeled and cut into large bite-sized pieces

50 ml/2 fl oz **whole milk**

1 teaspoon **Dijon mustard**

75 g/2½ oz **Cheddar cheese**, grated

Green vegetables, to serve

What to do

1. Heat the oil in a large saucepan over a medium–low heat. Add the swede or parsnip, carrots and leek, part-cover with a lid and cook for 15 minutes, stirring frequently, until softened. Add the garlic, tomatoes, lentils and herbs and cook for a further 10 minutes, part-covered, until the vegetables are tender.

2. Meanwhile, cook the potatoes in a large saucepan of boiling water for 12–15 minutes until tender. Drain, then return the potatoes to the pan with the milk, mustard and half the cheese. Mash until smooth.

3. Preheat the grill to high. Spoon the vegetable mixture into an ovenproof dish, top with the mash and scatter over the remaining cheese. Grill for 10 minutes, or until golden on top. Serve with green vegetables.

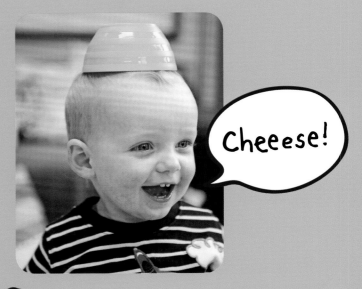

Cheeese!

Smelly socks!

Feed the senses

Dried herbs are brilliant for sniffing games. Put a teaspoon of dried mint, basil, oregano and mixed herbs in a baby sock (one herb per sock), then let your little one have a good sniff. Play a game matching up the smelly socks to the smells of the herbs in their pots.

Seaside carbonara

serves
2+2
adults + kids
prep
10 minutes
cook
15 minutes

This fishy twist on a carbonara uses canned salmon to make it super-easy to put together. Salmon has lots of healthy omega-3 fats to help oil your baby's developing brain. Clever!

What you need

280 g/10 oz dried **spaghetti**

1 **courgette**, diced

2 teaspoons **olive oil**

1 large **garlic** clove, finely chopped

350 g/12 oz canned **red salmon** in water, drained, any skin and bones removed and flesh flaked

100 ml/3½ fl oz **double cream**

50 ml/2 fl oz **whole milk**

Juice of ½ **lemon**

1 teaspoon finely grated **lemon** rind

2–3 tablespoons snipped **chives**

Freshly ground **black pepper**

What to do

1. Cook the pasta in a saucepan of boiling water according to the packet instructions until tender, adding the courgette 2 minutes before the end of the cooking time. Drain, reserving the cooking water. Return the pasta and courgette to the pan.

2. Meanwhile, heat the oil in a saucepan over a low heat and cook the garlic for 1 minute until softened, stirring and taking care not to let it brown. Stir in the salmon, then pour in the cream and milk and warm through for 5 minutes, stirring frequently.

3. Stir in the lemon juice, lemon rind and chives. Season with a little pepper and warm through gently. Pour the sauce over the pasta, add 4 tablespoons of the reserved cooking water and warm through over a low heat, tossing until combined. Finely chop the pasta for babies before serving.

Sea spaghetti

feed the senses

Try this sensorial activity with your baby. Cook up a bowl of spaghetti. Run it under cold water to stop it sticking and stir through plenty of oil to make it super-slimy. Add blue food colouring (use the non-staining sort) and stir away until all the spaghetti is blue. Pop in some fishy bathtime toys and encourage your little one to delve his or her hands into the slippery sea to find what's lurking beneath.

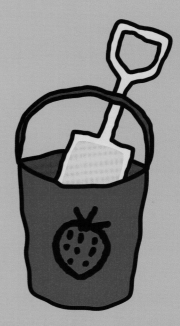

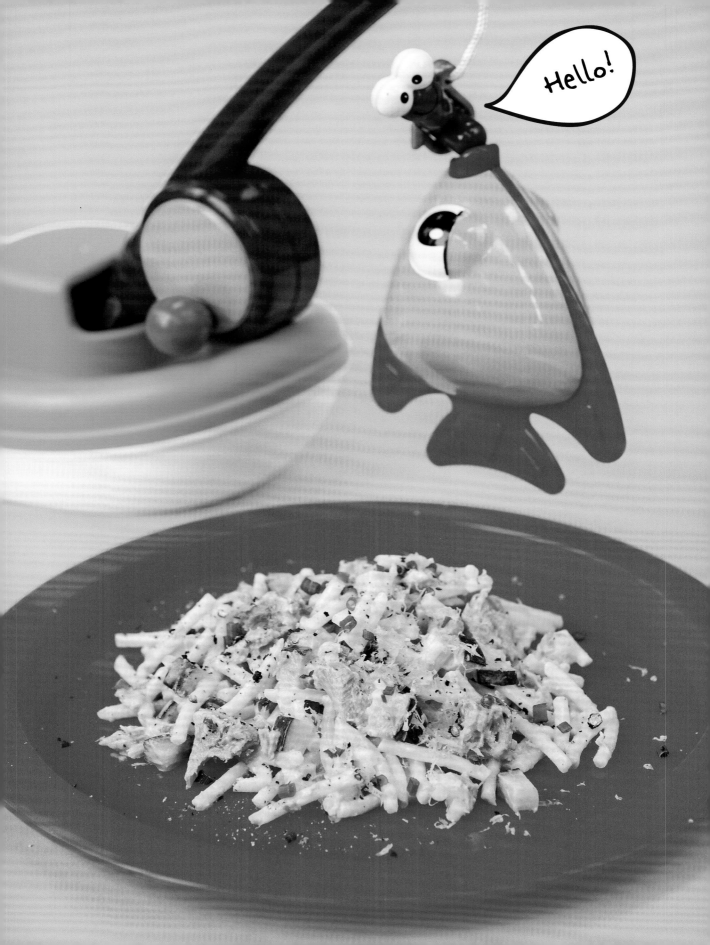

Sticky fingers BBQ chicken

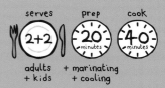

serves 2+2 adults + kids

prep 20 minutes + marinating + cooling

cook 40 minutes

The tangy sauce on this chicken will mean there's lots of finger-licking and lip-smacking at teatime. Little ones can help cut out their favourite polenta shapes for serving, too!

What you need

6 bone-in **chicken thighs** (about 800 g/1 lb 12 oz), skin trimmed

Olive oil, for greasing

Peas and **sweetcorn**, to serve

For the marinade

1 teaspoon **balsamic vinegar**

1 teaspoon reduced-salt **soy sauce**

1 tablespoon **clear honey**

1 tablespoon **tomato purée**

For the polenta shapes

115 g/4 oz **instant polenta**

30 g/1 oz **unsalted butter**

30 g/1 oz **Parmesan cheese**, finely grated

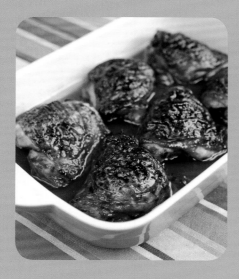

What to do

1. Mix together the ingredients for the marinade in a shallow, non-reactive dish. Make 3 cuts into the top of each chicken thigh, then place in the dish and spoon the marinade over until coated. Cover with clingfilm and leave to marinate in the fridge for at least 30 minutes.

2. Meanwhile, grease a small baking tray. Pour 575 ml/18 fl oz water into a saucepan and place over a medium heat. Gradually pour in the polenta and cook for 8–10 minutes, stirring continuously, until smooth and thick. Stir in the butter and Parmesan until combined. Transfer the polenta to the prepared baking tray, then smooth it out in an even layer about 1 cm/½ inch thick. Leave to cool and firm up.

3. Preheat the oven to 200°C/400°F/Gas Mark 6. Lightly oil a large, nonstick roasting tin. Place the chicken in the tin, spooning over any remaining marinade from the dish. Bake in the oven for 25–30 minutes, or until the juices run clear when the thickest part of the chicken is pierced with a sharp knife.

4. Meanwhile, using your favourite dough cutter, stamp out shapes in the polenta. Heat a large, nonstick frying pan and brush with oil, then fry the polenta shapes for 3–4 minutes on each side until slightly crisp and golden.

5. Remove the meat from the bones for the children's portions and finely chop, then serve with the polenta shapes, peas and sweetcorn.

Softly spiced chicken + sultana curry

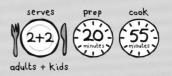

serves **2+2** adults + kids

prep **20** minutes

cook **55** minutes

Adventurous taste buds will love the sweet and spicy ginger in this curry and the burst of sweetness from the sultanas. Ginger is especially gentle for your baby's delicate little tummy.

What you need

1 tablespoon **sunflower oil**

4 skinless, boneless **chicken thighs** (about 400 g/14 oz), each cut into five strips

1 large **onion**, finely sliced

1 **garlic** clove, finely chopped

4 cm/1½ inch piece of fresh **root ginger**, peeled and finely chopped

1 tablespoon **mild or medium curry powder**

1 tablespoon **garam masala**

400 g/14 oz can **chopped tomatoes**

A large handful of **coriander** leaves, finely chopped

50 g/1¾ oz **sultanas**

200 ml/7 fl oz **natural yogurt**

Rice and **green vegetables**, to serve

What to do

1. Heat the oil in a saucepan over a medium heat and cook the chicken, in 2 batches, for 5 minutes until browned all over. Remove with a slotted spoon and set aside.

2. Reduce the heat to medium–low, add the onion to the pan and cook for 5 minutes, stirring frequently, until softened. Add the garlic, ginger, curry powder and garam masala and cook for a further 2 minutes, stirring.

3. Return the chicken to the pan with the tomatoes, coriander and sultanas, part-cover with a lid and simmer gently for 30 minutes until the chicken is cooked through and the sauce has reduced and thickened.

4. Reduce the heat to low and stir in the yogurt. Cook for a further 5 minutes, stirring occasionally, until heated through. Finely chop the chicken for babies, then serve with rice and green vegetables.

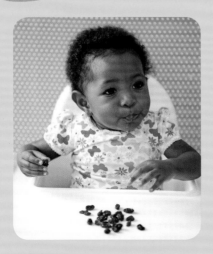

Feed the senses

Veggie treasure

Dried rice feels lovely against little fingers. Hide some raw broccoli florets in a deep tub filled with rice and encourage your little one to feel around for the veggie treasure. Put a cloth on the floor to catch any grains that spill out!

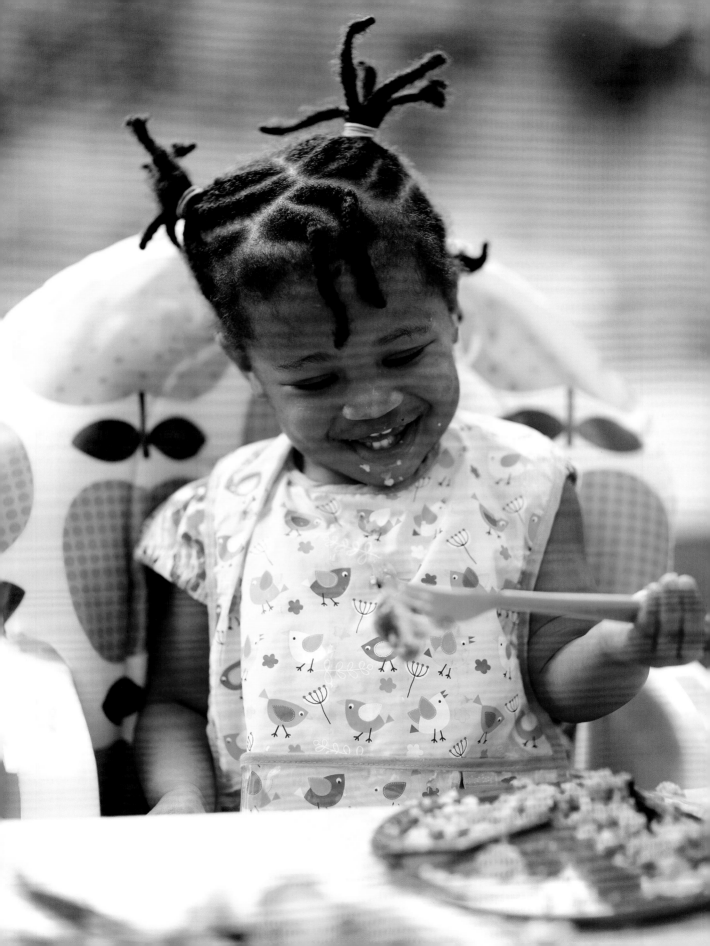

Baked + bursting butternut squash

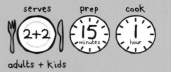

serves 2+2 adults + kids | prep 15 minutes | cook 1 hour

This is a dish the whole family will love. It's bursting with yumminess, as well as the goodness of vitamin A, which will help to make little eyes healthy.

What you need

1 large **butternut squash**, halved lengthways and deseeded

1 tablespoon **olive oil**

1 **leek**, trimmed, cleaned and finely chopped

1 **courgette**, finely chopped

2 teaspoons **thyme** leaves or 1 teaspoon **dried thyme**

40 g/1½ oz **pine nuts**, finely chopped

15 g/½ oz **Parmesan cheese**, finely grated

10 g/¼ oz **Cheddar cheese**, finely grated

Green vegetables and **rice** or **couscous**, to serve

What to do

1. Preheat the oven to 200°C/400°F/Gas Mark 6. Place the squash in a roasting tin, cut sides up, and brush the tops with 1 teaspoon of the oil. Roast for 45 minutes, or until tender.

2. Meanwhile, heat the remaining oil in a small, nonstick frying pan over a medium–low heat and cook the leek and courgette for 5 minutes, stirring frequently, until softened. Stir in the thyme and pine nuts. Tip into a large bowl.

3. Scoop the squash flesh into the leek mixture, then using the back of a fork mash together to a coarse purée. Spoon the mixture into the squash skins, sprinkle the cheeses over the top and roast for a further 15 minutes until golden.

4. Scoop out the children's portions, then serve with green vegetables and rice or couscous.

Leaf picking

Can I help?

Encourage your little one to perfect that pincer grip by asking for help picking the tiny thyme leaves from the stalks.

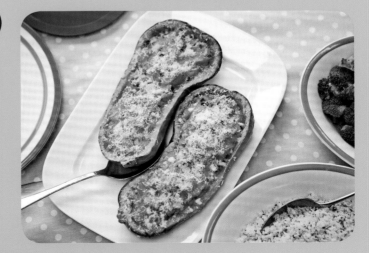

129

Sunshine chicken with mushy minty peas

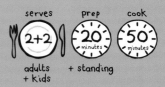

serves 2+2 adults + kids | prep 20 minutes + standing | cook 50 minutes

Peas and mint give this chicken-and-rice dish a delicious, summer freshness – and add a hint of green. Why not dine al fresco and imagine you're on a summer holiday?

What you need

1 tablespoon **olive oil**

1 large **onion**, chopped

4 skinless, boneless **chicken thighs** (about 400 g/14 oz), cut into bite-sized pieces

2 **garlic** cloves, chopped

225 g/8 oz **brown rice**

575 ml/18 fl oz **chicken stock**

1 large **leek**, trimmed, cleaned and sliced

100 g/3½ oz **frozen peas**

A handful of **mint** leaves, finely chopped, plus extra to serve

15 g/½ oz **unsalted butter**

Parmesan cheese, finely grated, to serve (optional)

What to do

1. Heat the oil in a large, heavy-based saucepan over a medium heat and cook the onion for 8 minutes, stirring frequently, until softened. Remove with a slotted spoon and set aside. Add half the chicken to the pan and cook for 5 minutes until browned all over. Remove with the slotted spoon and set aside, then cook the remaining chicken.

2. Return the onion and the first batch of chicken to the pan with the garlic and rice and stir until combined. Pour in the stock, stir well and bring to the boil, then reduce the heat to its lowest setting, cover with a lid and simmer for 25 minutes until the rice is tender, the stock is absorbed and the chicken is cooked through. Stir occasionally to prevent it sticking and add a little boiled water if necessary.

3. Meanwhile, steam or boil the leek and peas over a medium heat for 5 minutes until tender. Purée the veg with the mint and 1 tablespoon of boiled water in a food processor, or using a hand blender, until smooth.

4. Stir the purée into the rice mixture, then turn off the heat. Stir in the butter, cover with a lid and leave to stand for 3 minutes. Finely chop the chicken for babies, then serve with extra mint and sprinkled with Parmesan, if using.

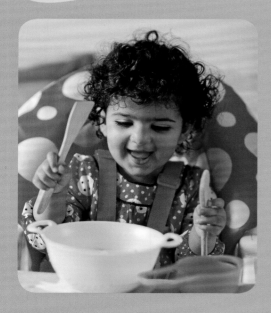

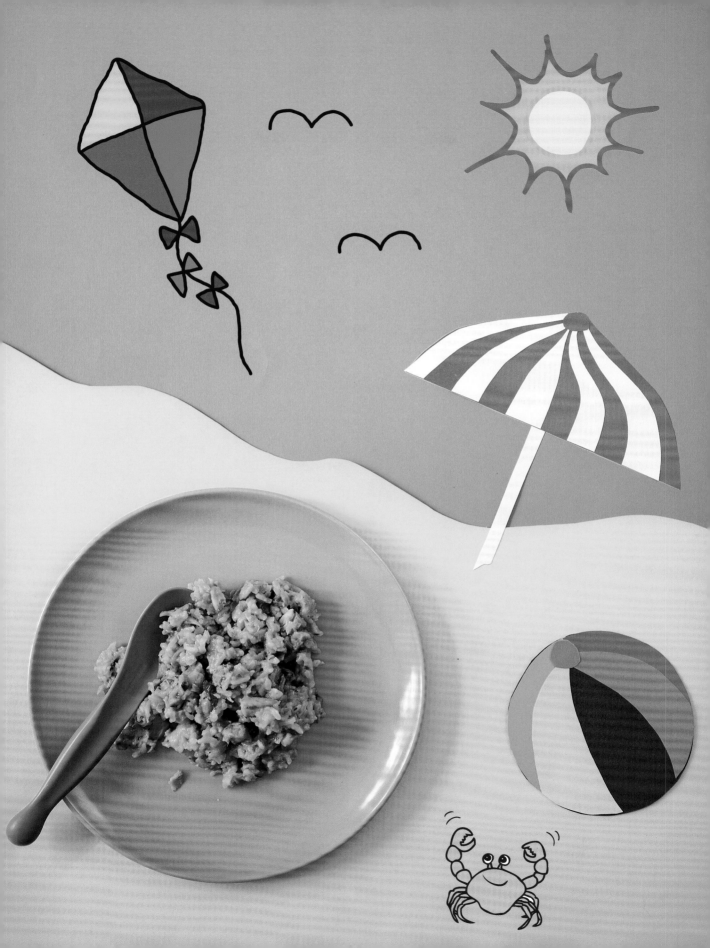

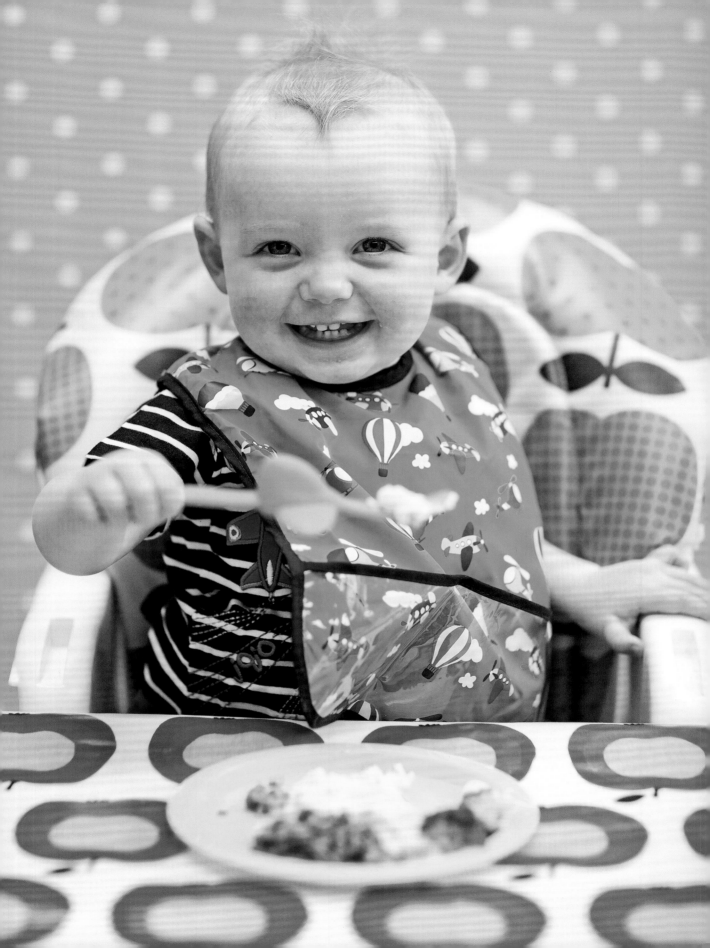

Perfect pair apple + pork ragù

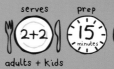

serves 2+2 adults + kids · prep 15 minutes · cook 1⅓ hours

When it comes to culinary harmony, pork and apple are the best of friends. Savoury and sweet, together they give your baby a punchy taste sensation that's just perfect.

What you need

600 g/1 lb 5 oz **pork shoulder steaks**, excess fat removed, cut into large bite-sized chunks

2 tablespoons **plain flour**

4 teaspoons **olive oil**

1 large **onion**, chopped

2 large **garlic** cloves, finely chopped

2 teaspoons **dried thyme**

275 ml/9 fl oz **chicken stock**

1 teaspoon **cider vinegar**

1 teaspoon **Dijon mustard**

1 **eating apple**, quartered, cored and cut into wedges

2 tablespoons **crème fraîche**

Mashed potato and **vegetables**, to serve

What to do

1. Preheat the oven to 180°C/350°F/Gas Mark 4. Toss the pork in the flour and set aside.

2. Heat half the oil in a large casserole dish over a medium heat. Add the onion, cover with a lid and cook for 5 minutes, stirring frequently, until softened. Remove with a slotted spoon and set aside.

3. Add the remaining oil to the pan, add half the pork and cook for 5 minutes, turning occasionally, until browned all over. Remove with the slotted spoon and set aside. Repeat with the remaining pork.

4. Return the first batch of pork and the onion to the pan and add the garlic and thyme. Stir until combined, then pour in the stock and vinegar. Bring to the boil, stirring to remove any bits from the bottom of the casserole. Stir in the mustard and add the apple.

5. Cover the casserole with a lid and bake in the oven for 50–60 minutes, stirring occasionally, until the pork is cooked through and tender. Remove from the oven and stir in the crème fraîche. Finely chop the pork for babies, then serve with mash and vegetables.

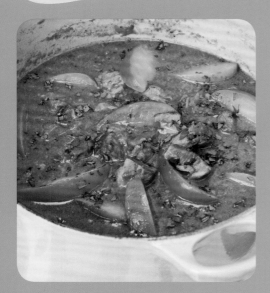

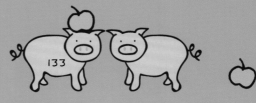

133

Lovely little mackerel salad

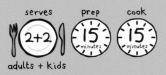

serves 2+2 adults + kids | prep 15 minutes | cook 15 minutes

Our little-one-friendly take on a Niçoise salad is crammed with goodness – the tomatoes give antioxidants, the mackerel gives healthy fats... and the generous olives give both! Try letting your baby pick up the pieces to taste each ingredient one by one.

What you need

280 g/10 oz **new potatoes**, halved

3 **eggs**

50 g/1¾ oz **green beans**, trimmed and very thinly sliced diagonally

140 g/5 oz **cherry tomatoes**, halved or quartered if large

40 g/1½ oz **pitted black or green olives** (not in brine), halved

110 g/3¾ oz can **grilled mackerel fillets**, skin and bones removed and flesh flaked

For the dressing (optional)

4 teaspoons **extra virgin olive oil**

4 teaspoons **lemon juice**

2 tablespoons **natural yogurt**

What to do

1. Cook the potatoes in a large saucepan of boiling water for 12–15 minutes until tender, adding the eggs 10 minutes and the beans 5 minutes before the end of the cooking time. Drain, then cool the beans and eggs under cold running water. Peel off the potato skins, if you prefer.

2. Cut the potatoes into bite-sized pieces and place in a serving bowl with the beans, tomatoes, olives and mackerel. Turn gently until combined. Shell the eggs and cut into wedges, then place on top of the salad.

3. For the dressing (if using), mix together the oil and lemon juice until combined, then stir in the yogurt. Spoon it over the salad before serving. Finely chop the salad for babies, or serve as finger food without dressing.

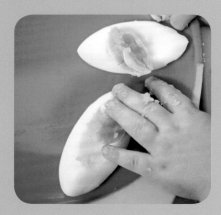

Can I help?

Stir it up

The sooner little ones can start to help in the kitchen, the better! See if your baby will help you stir the dressing ingredients and then pour them over the salad.

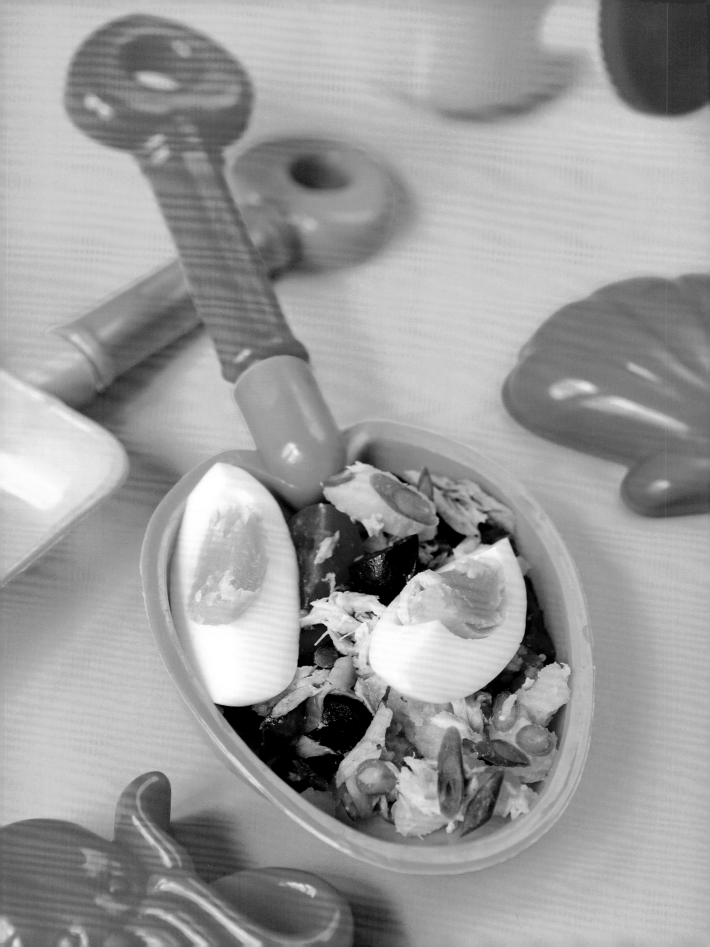

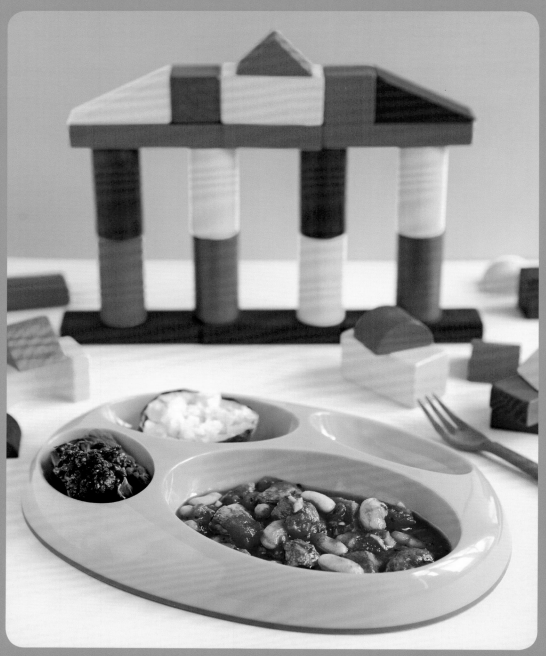

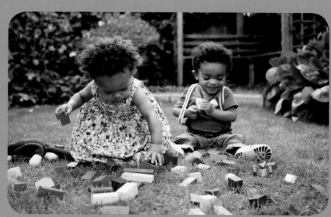

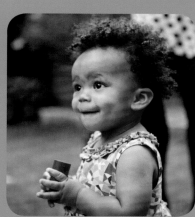

Go Greek lamb stew

Little ones could try building their own temple while this slow-cooked Greek stew bubbles away. Cinnamon and cloves make it warm, just like Greek sunshine.

What you need

1 tablespoon **olive oil**

1 large **onion**, chopped

600 g/1 lb 5 oz diced **shoulder or leg of lamb**, excess fat removed

3 **garlic** cloves, finely chopped

1 small **cinnamon stick**

6 **cloves**

1 teaspoon **dried oregano**

2 tablespoons **red wine vinegar**

400 g/14 oz can **chopped tomatoes**

2 tablespoons **tomato purée**

150 g/5½ oz canned **cannellini beans** in water, drained and rinsed

Baked potatoes and **favourite veggies**, to serve

What to do

1. Preheat the oven to 170°C/325°F/Gas Mark 3. Heat the oil in a large casserole over a medium heat. Add the onion, cover with a lid and cook for 8 minutes, stirring occasionally, until softened. Remove with a slotted spoon and set aside.

2. Add half the lamb to the pan and cook for 5 minutes until browned all over. Remove with the slotted spoon and set aside. Repeat with the remaining lamb.

3. Return the onion and the first batch of lamb to the pan with the garlic, cinnamon, cloves and oregano. Stir well and add the vinegar, chopped tomatoes and tomato purée. Pour in 150 ml/¼ pint water, stir in the beans and bring to the boil.

4. Cover the casserole with the lid and bake in the oven for 1½ hours, or until the lamb is tender. (Cook the baked potatoes at the same time.) Check the stew halfway through cooking to make sure it's not dry, adding a little extra water if necessary.

5. Remove the cinnamon stick, then finely chop the stew for babies. Serve with half a baked potato and favourite veggies.

Our friends say...

'I love meals such as stews and casseroles that I can cook in my slow cooker. I put all the ingredients in at breakfast time and then – like magic – by teatime, a perfect meal!'

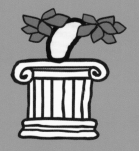

Chicken paella-ella-ella

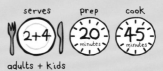

serves 2+4 adults + kids
prep 20 minutes
cook 45 minutes

The rainbow of colours in this paella shows that it bursts with goodness. Get your streamers ready – this is a one-pot meal sure to create a carnival mood in your kitchen!

What you need

1 tablespoon **olive oil**

2 **unsmoked bacon rashers**, cut into small pieces

4 skinless, boneless **chicken thighs** (about 400 g/14 oz), cut into bite-sized pieces

1 **onion**, finely chopped

1 small **red pepper**, cored, deseeded and chopped

2 **garlic** cloves, finely chopped

225 g/8 oz **paella rice**

A large pinch of **saffron threads** or 1 teaspoon **turmeric**

1 heaped teaspoon **smoked paprika**

1 teaspoon **dried thyme**

725 ml/1¼ pints hot **chicken stock**

100 g/3½ oz **frozen petits pois**

4 **tomatoes**, deseeded and diced

Juice of ½ **lemon**

What to do

1. Heat the oil in a large, nonstick frying pan over a medium heat and cook the bacon for 5 minutes until almost crisp, then remove with a slotted spoon. Add the chicken to the pan, in 2 batches, and cook each batch for 5 minutes until the chicken is browned all over. Remove with the slotted spoon and set aside.

2. Reduce the heat slightly, add the onion and red pepper to the pan and cook for 5 minutes, stirring frequently, until softened. Add the garlic and return the bacon and chicken to the pan with the rice. Stir until combined.

3. Mix the saffron or turmeric, paprika and thyme into the hot stock and pour it into the pan. Bring to the boil, then reduce the heat and simmer for 15 minutes, without stirring. Add the petits pois and tomatoes, press them into the rice and cook for a further 10 minutes, or until the chicken is cooked through and the rice is tender. Pour over the lemon juice, cover and leave to stand for 5 minutes. Finely chop the paella for babies before serving.

Have a carnival!

Just for fun

Eating together is the perfect reason to celebrate – turn teatime into a family festival. Find whistles and blowers and make some noise! Make sure everyone has a party hat, too!

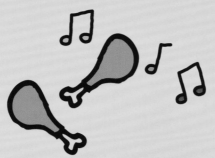

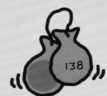

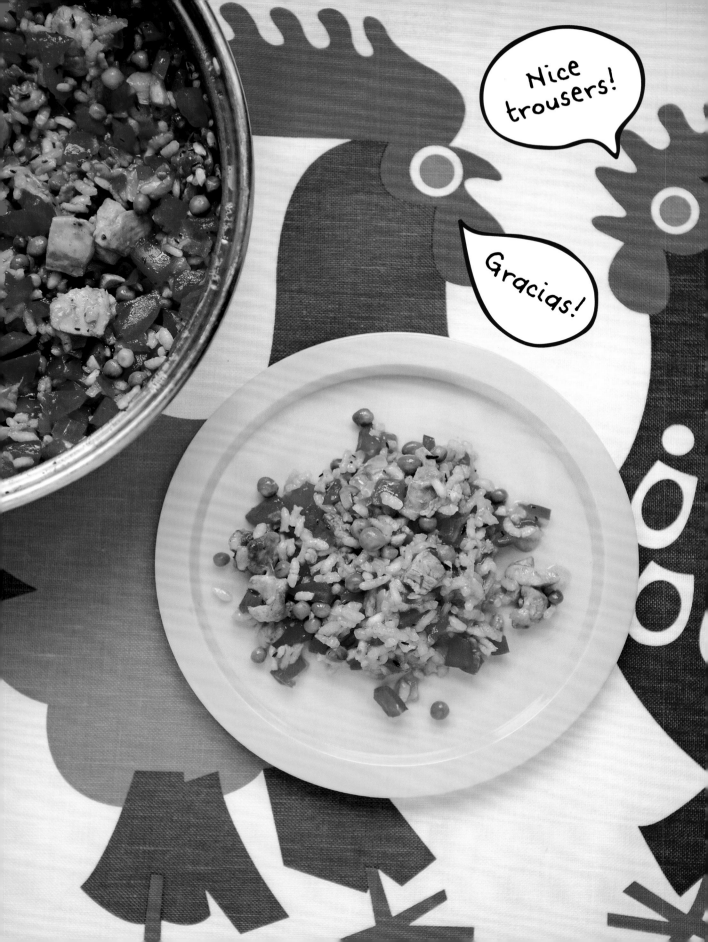

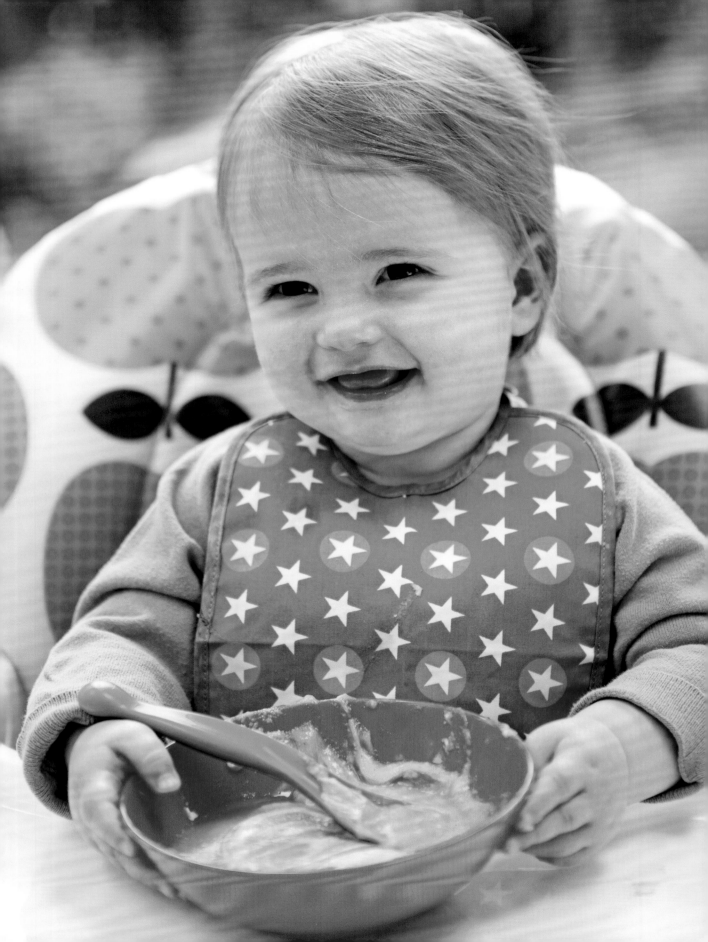

Speedy spiced lentil soup

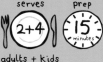

serves 2+4 adults + kids | prep 15 minutes | cook 20 minutes

This is possibly the quickest lentil soup we've ever made! For a thicker consistency that's easier for little ones to keep on the spoon, add less water. *Slurrrp.*

What you need

150 g/5½ oz dried **split red lentils**, rinsed

1 **onion**, finely chopped

1 large **carrot**, peeled and sliced

1 large **potato** (about 280 g/ 10 oz), peeled and cut into bite-sized pieces

900 ml/1½ pints **vegetable stock**

2 **bay leaves**

1 tablespoon **mild curry powder**

Hummus, to serve (optional; see pp.166–7)

What to do

1. Place the lentils, onion, carrot, potato, stock and bay leaves in a large saucepan and bring to the boil. Reduce the heat, part-cover with a lid and simmer for 12 minutes, skimming off any foam that rises to the surface. Stir in the curry powder and cook for a further 3 minutes until everything is tender.

2. Remove the bay leaves, then purée in a food processor or using a hand blender. Serve topped with a spoonful of hummus, if using.

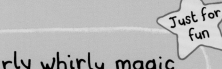

Swirly whirly magic

Hold a spoon in your little one's hand and together create a swirly whirly pattern in the hummus topping. Then, mix it up quickly and watch it disappear like magic.

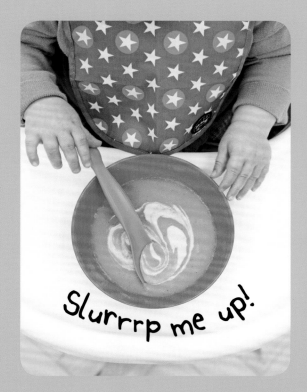

Slurrrp me up!

Slowly-does-it beef stew + dumplings

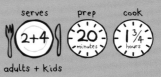

serves
2+4
adults + kids

prep
20 minutes

cook
1 3/4 hours

Fill up hungry tummies with this warming beef-and-veg stew. The cheesy dumplings are optional, but we like to serve them on the side for little hands to dunk. Splosh!

What you need

1 tablespoon **olive oil**

2 **onions**, roughly chopped

600 g/1 lb 5 oz diced **lean braising or stewing steak**, excess fat removed

2 tablespoons **plain flour**

200 g/7 oz **mushrooms**, chopped

3 **carrots**, peeled and thickly sliced

2 **turnips**, peeled and diced

1 **bay leaf**

½ teaspoon **thyme** leaves

900 ml/1½ pints **beef stock**

1 teaspoon **English mustard**

1 teaspoon **balsamic vinegar**

For the cheesy dumplings

100 g/3½ oz **plain flour**

50 g/1¾ oz **suet**

1 tablespoon **thyme** leaves

30 g/1 oz **Cheddar cheese**, grated

What to do

1. Heat the oil in a large casserole over a medium heat and cook the onions for 5 minutes, stirring frequently, until softened. Remove with a slotted spoon and set aside.

2. Toss the beef in the flour until coated all over, then add half to the casserole and cook for 5 minutes until browned all over. Remove with the slotted spoon and set aside. Repeat with the remaining beef.

3. Return the onions and the first batch of beef to the pan with the mushrooms, carrots, turnips, bay leaf, thyme and stock. Bring to the boil, then reduce the heat to low, part-cover with a lid and cook for 1¼ hours, stirring occasionally, until reduced and thickened. Stir in the mustard and vinegar.

4. Meanwhile, make the dumplings. Place the flour in a bowl and rub in the suet until combined. Stir in the thyme and cheese with 5–6 tablespoons of water to make a stiff dough. Divide into 8 equal pieces and shape into dumplings. Arrange on top of the stew, cover with the lid and cook for a further 20 minutes until the dumplings are risen and fluffy and the beef is tender. Finely chop the stew and dumplings for babies before serving; or serve the dumplings as a finger food on the side.

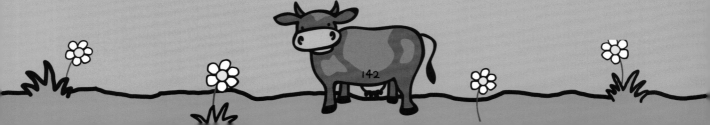

Catch-of-the-day spag bol

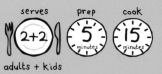

serves 2+2 adults + kids | prep 5 minutes | cook 15 minutes

Canned tuna makes a scrummy alternative to the beef mince you'd usually find in bolognese. We think you'll love it so much, you'll make it a favourite for the whole family.

What you need

280 g/10 oz dried **spaghetti**

1 **carrot**, peeled and diced

1 tablespoon **olive oil**

2 **garlic** cloves, finely chopped

1 teaspoon **dried oregano**

400 g/14 oz can **chopped tomatoes**

2 tablespoons **tomato purée**

200 g /7 oz can **tuna chunks** in spring water, drained

Broccoli, to serve

What to do

1. Cook the pasta in a saucepan of boiling water according to the packet instructions until tender, adding the carrot 8 minutes before the end of the cooking time. Drain, reserving the cooking water.

2. Meanwhile, place the oil and garlic in a nonstick frying pan over a medium–low heat and cook for 1 minute. Add the oregano, tomatoes and tomato purée and cook for a further 8 minutes, stirring frequently.

3. Stir in the tuna, breaking it up slightly, and cook for 2 minutes, then add the pasta, carrot and 4 tablespoons of the reserved cooking water and heat through. Finely chop the pasta for babies, then serve with broccoli.

Our friends say...

'I show my little one the whole vegetables I'm cooking with. I hand her a carrot, say, and let her hold, feel and smell it. Then, I show her how I peel and chop it and make it yummy for her to eat. When she's older, she can gnaw on a raw bit as I cook, too.'

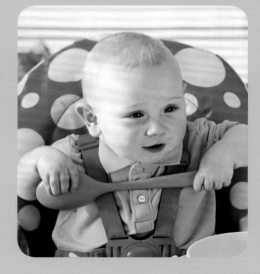

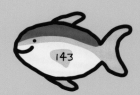

Big veg chunky chilli

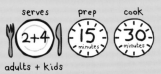

serves 2+4 adults + kids | prep 15 minutes | cook 30 minutes

We've put just enough chilli in this dish to excite budding taste adventurers – but if your little one is showing signs of a fiery palate, by all means spice it up with a teaspoon more.

What you need

450 g/1 lb **butternut squash**, peeled, deseeded and cut into large bite-sized pieces

1 tablespoon **olive oil**

100 g/3½ oz **mushrooms**, sliced

2 **garlic** cloves, finely chopped

400 ml/14 fl oz **passata** (sieved tomatoes)

2 tablespoons **tomato purée**

400 g/14 oz can **red kidney beans** in water, drained

4 **cloves**

1 teaspoon **ground ginger**

1 teaspoon **mild chilli powder**

Brown rice and **green vegetables**, to serve

What to do

1. Preheat the oven to 180°C/350°F/Gas Mark 4. Toss the squash in half the oil, then spread it out in a roasting tray and roast in the oven for 30 minutes, turning once, until tender and slightly golden.

2. Meanwhile, heat the remaining oil in a large saucepan over a medium heat and cook the mushrooms for 6 minutes, stirring frequently, until softened. Stir in the garlic, then add the passata, tomato purée, beans, cloves, ginger and chilli powder and bring almost to the boil. Reduce the heat, part-cover with a lid and simmer for 15 minutes until reduced and thickened. Add a splash of water if the sauce is too thick.

3. When the squash is cooked, stir it into the chilli. Finely chop the chilli for babies, then serve with rice and green vegetables.

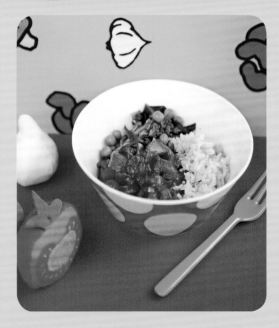

Scoop the seeds

Just for fun

Use an ice-cream scoop to remove the seeds from the squash – it's so quick and easy! And don't forget to save the seeds to use in a shaker for your baby, or as counting beans for toddlers.

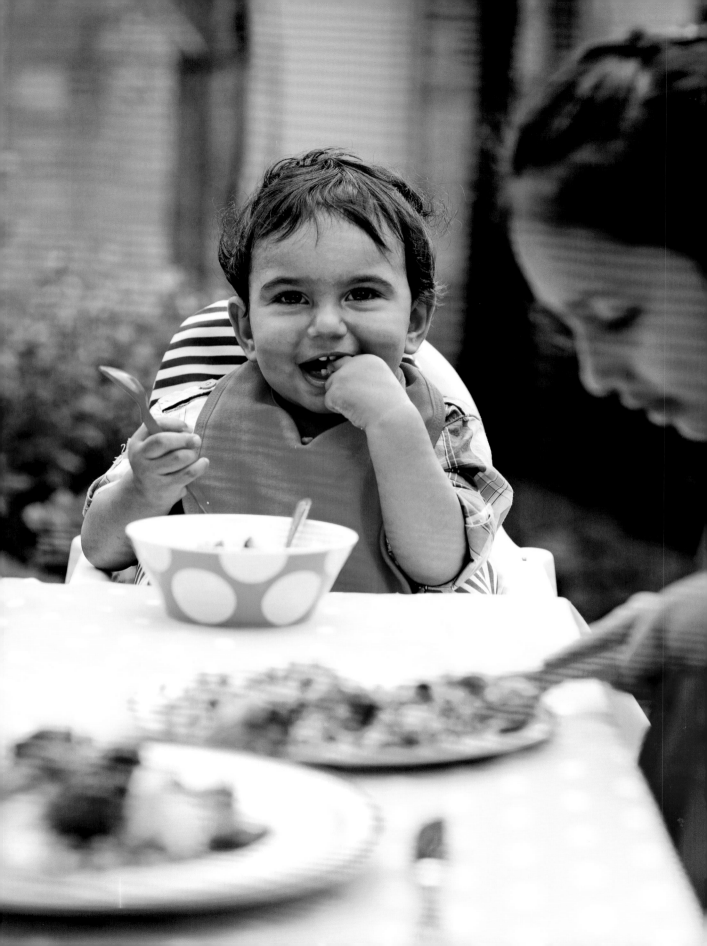

All-for-me apple crumbles

makes **4** · prep **15** minutes · cook **30** minutes

We love these simple crumbles. Cut the apples in half, top them with crumble and bake them just as they are. Virtually instant deliciousness!

What you need

2 **eating apples**, halved horizontally

For the crumble mix

40 g/1½ oz **plain flour**

30 g/1 oz chilled **unsalted butter**, cubed, plus extra for greasing

1 ripe **banana**, finely chopped

1 teaspoon **ground cinnamon**

1 tablespoon **sunflower seeds**, finely chopped

2 tablespoons **porridge oats**

What to do

1) Preheat the oven to 190°C/375°F/Gas Mark 5. To make the crumble mix, place the flour in a bowl, add the butter and rub in with your fingertips until the mixture resembles coarse breadcrumbs. Stir in the banana, cinnamon, seeds and oats.

2) Using a teaspoon, scoop out the core from each apple half. Rub a little butter over the top of each half and sprinkle the crumble mixture over. Place the apples in a small roasting tin, packing them tightly together, and add 1 tablespoon of water to the tin. Bake in the oven for 25–30 minutes until the apples are tender and the crumble is crisp.

Rub-a-dub-dub

Can I help?

When you're little, what could be better than squishing together butter and flour? Let your little one have a go at making crumble. Oooo... messy fingers!

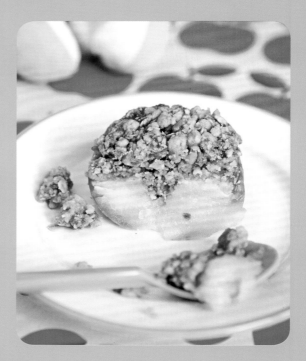

Deliciously sticky date squares

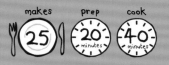

makes **25** · prep **20** minutes · cook **40** minutes

These squares are *reeeally* sticky! But they're also full of goodness. Dates are rich in fibre and packed with iron, so this little treat is a real goody two shoes!

What you need

175 g/6 oz **unsalted butter**, melted, plus extra for greasing

1 large **cooking apple** (about 150 g/5½ oz), peeled, cored and diced

150 g/5½ oz **pitted dried dates**

200 g/7 oz **plain flour**

100 g/3½ oz **soft light brown sugar**

1 teaspoon **bicarbonate of soda**

75 g/2½ oz **porridge oats**

What to do

1. Preheat the oven to 190°C/375°F/Gas Mark 5. Lightly grease a 23 cm/9 inch square cake tin and line the base with baking parchment.

2. Place the apple, dates and 175 ml/6 fl oz water in a saucepan, cover with a lid and cook over a low heat for 15 minutes, stirring occasionally, until softened. Using the back of a fork, mash the fruit until smooth.

3. Meanwhile, mix together the flour, sugar, bicarbonate of soda and porridge oats in a large bowl. Pour in the melted butter and mix everything together.

4. Spoon two-thirds of the mixture into the prepared tin and press down firmly in an even layer. Spread the apple mixture evenly over the top to cover. Sprinkle the remaining oat mixture over the top and bake in the oven for 25 minutes until cooked through and just starting to turn golden. Mark into 25 squares while still warm, then leave to cool in the tin. Cut fully into the squares and store in an airtight container for up to 4 days.

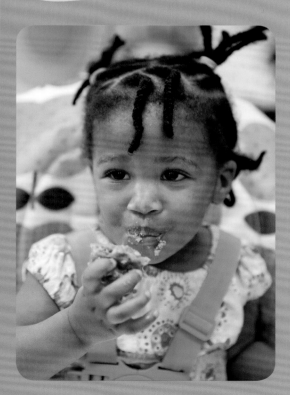

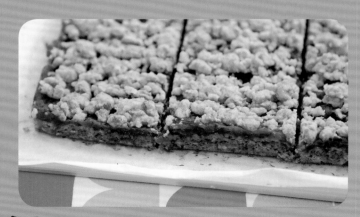

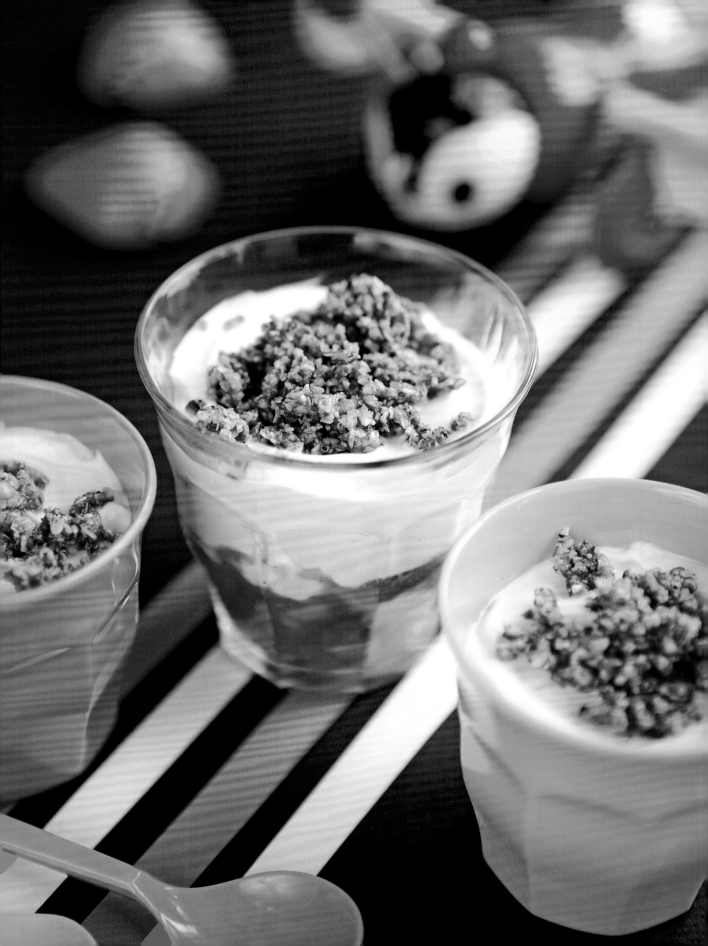

Stripy berry puds

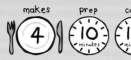

makes **4** | prep **10** minutes | cook **10** minutes

There are three layers of scrumminess in this perfect pudding – a fruity bottom, a creamy middle and a crunchy top! Let little ones help build their own to practise their spoon skills.

What you need

20 g/¾ oz **pecan nut halves**

1 tablespoon **sunflower seeds**

3 tablespoons **porridge oats**

2 teaspoons **clear honey**

250 g/9 oz **strawberries** or **your favourite berries**, hulled

1 teaspoon **vanilla extract**

250 ml/9 fl oz **thick natural yogurt**

What to do

1. Place the pecans and sunflower seeds in a large, nonstick frying pan over a medium–low heat and dry-fry for 3–4 minutes, turning occasionally, until slightly browned. Keep an eye on them as they can easily burn. Remove from the pan and finely chop, then tip into a bowl and leave to cool.

2. Add the oats to the pan and dry-fry over a medium–low heat for 3–4 minutes, turning occasionally, until toasted and slightly browned. Tip into the bowl with the pecans and leave to cool. Stir in the honey until everything is coated.

3. Purée 50 g/2 oz of the strawberries in a food processor, or using a hand blender, then stir in the vanilla extract. Finely chop the remaining strawberries and stir them into the purée. Divide the strawberry mixture equally between 4 glasses. Top with yogurt and then the oat mixture just before serving. (You may have some of the oat mixture left over; store it in an airtight container for up to 3 days.)

Ella's shortcut

You can use any of your favourite Ella's Kitchen fruit pouches to make these puds – we love apples, apples, apples or pears, pears, pears or bananas, bananas, bananas!

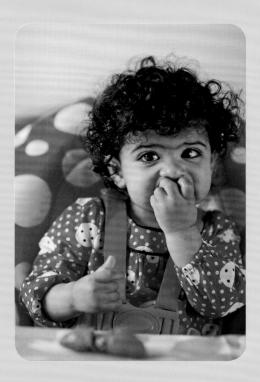

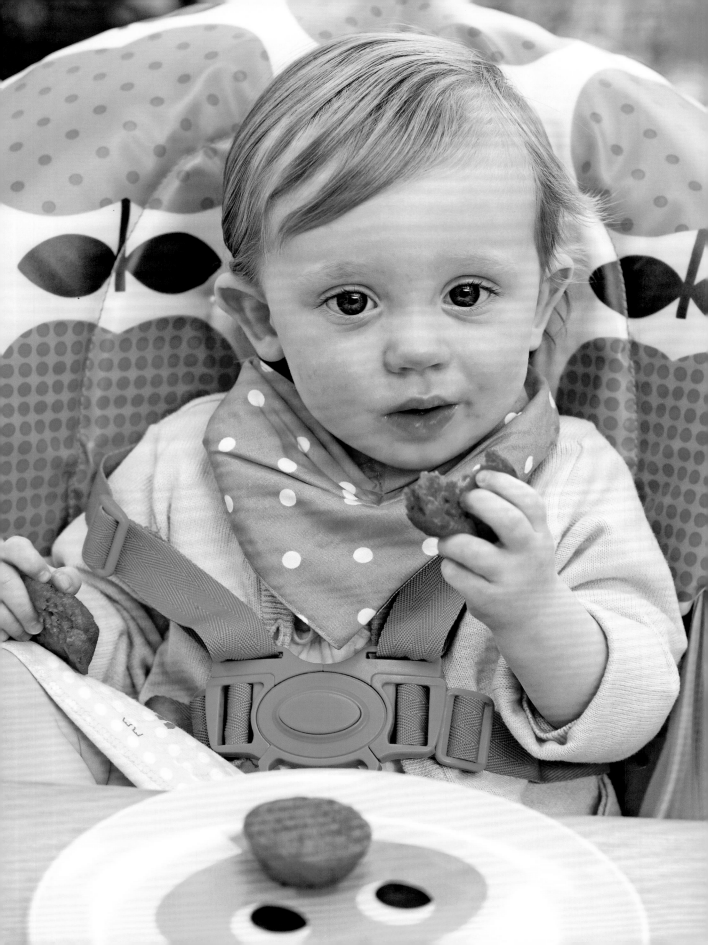

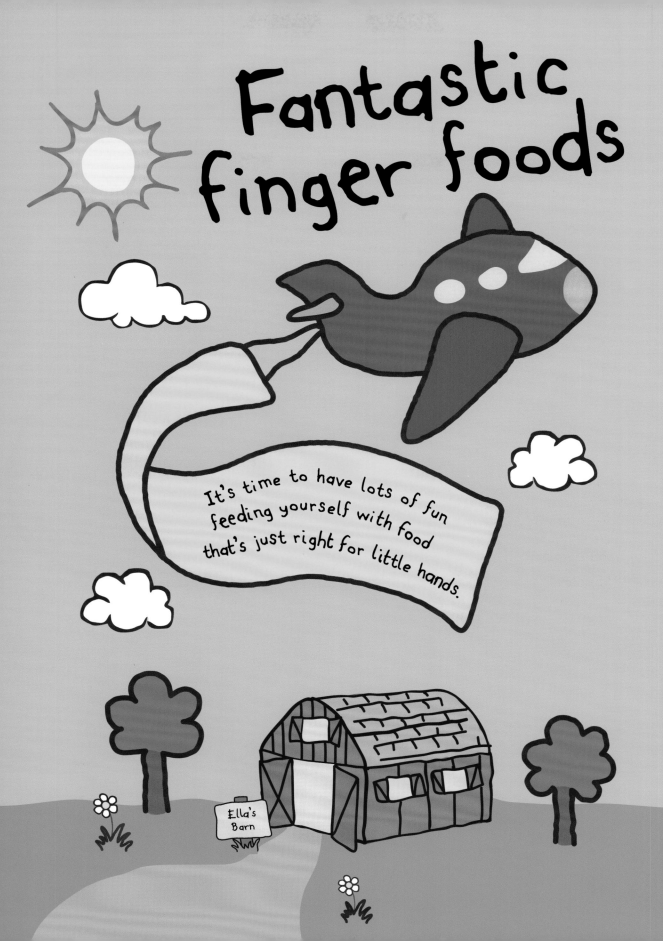

Finger foods for every day

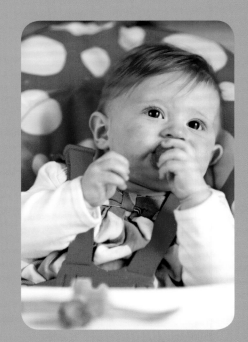

Babies' instincts are to bring whatever is in reach to their mouths – which means it makes sense to offer foods they can pick up. Organized age by age from 7 months, this chapter is packed with delicious finger foods that give your baby a little bit of foody independence.

Thumbs up for finger foods

Finger foods are a brilliant way for babies to practise hand–eye coordination (they have to concentrate really hard to get something into their open mouths without missing), and to tingle the touch sensors on tiny fingers.

Most of all, though, as they grow, babies love to feel that they have some influence over their world – it makes them feel *reeeally* good if they can do little things for themselves. Finger foods are the perfect opportunity for baby-style DIY!

Our friends say...

'I was so worried about my baby choking on her finger foods that I signed up for a first-aid course. I think it's a really good idea to go online or do a course to learn what to do in the event of choking – if only for peace of mind.'

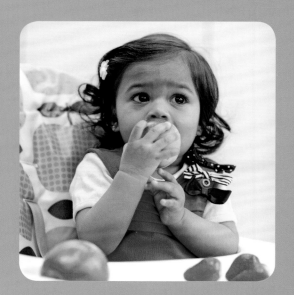

What to give

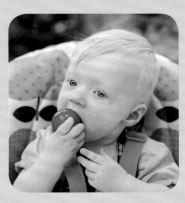

At 6 months finger foods must be super-soft and mush down easily, so they practically melt in your baby's mouth. Try well-cooked soft veg (such as batons of cooked carrot, parsnip or swede) and pieces of soft fruit (such as slices of banana, melon or peeled peach).

At 7 months, when babies' gums start to toughen up, try soft pieces of food now with a little texture. Toasted, crustless bread soldiers are perfect.

At 10 months finger foods can start to be a little firmer, especially if your baby has a few teeth. Thinner, flatter strips of food are good now, to help your baby's budding pincer grip – but avoid crumbly, flaky or brittle textures. Cooked strips of soft, moist meat, strips of well-cooked omelette, and cooked pasta shapes are all good choices.

From 12 months finger foods can become much smaller – older babies usually have a good pincer grip and are able to pick things up between thumb and forefinger. Soft foods are still best – we like chopped-up pieces of strawberry and halved or quartered grapes (not whole until your baby is at least 3 years old), small cubes of cheese, and little meatballs or falafels (see p.180).

Staying safe

We want to make sure your baby is completely safe at all times, so here's some info about gagging and choking so that you can spot the signs and know when to act.

Gagging It's perfectly normal for babies to gag as soft, little pieces of food move to the back of their tongues. It can be quite scary to watch, but a baby's gagging reflex is far more sensitive than an adult's. Through gagging, your baby's clever body moves the food forward for another go at chewing, or for spitting out. Try not to worry – keep smiling, and reassure your baby that everything is okay.

Choking This happens when a piece of food has slipped down and got stuck in your baby's windpipe (talk to your health visitor about what to do in this scenario). To prevent choking, never leave your baby alone while eating and never offer any food that could be a choking risk. Avoid popcorn, undercooked vegetables, frankfurters, whole grapes and cherries (or other fruit and veg with 'shiny' skins), and large pieces of banana until your baby reaches at least 3 years old; and avoid whole nuts until your little one is 5.

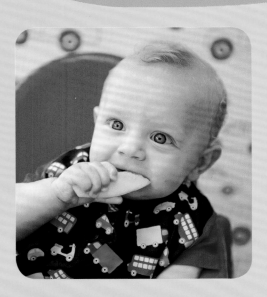

153

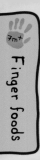
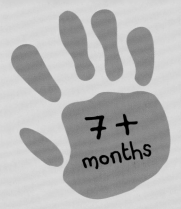

7 + months

By 7 months old your little taste explorers will be picking up pieces of fruit and other chunky finger foods in their fists and bringing them to their mouths. Yippeee!

Easy-cheesy eggy bread

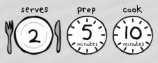

serves **2** | prep **5** minutes | cook **10** minutes

This cheesy twist on eggy bread is perfect for breakfast – or lunch or tea! Make sure the fingers have cooled enough for little hands to hold.

What you need

- 1 **egg**, lightly beaten
- 2 tablespoons **baby's usual milk**
- 10 g/¼ oz **Parmesan cheese**, finely grated
- 1 slice of **thick wholemeal bread**
- 10 g/¼ oz **unsalted butter**

What to do

1. Mix together the egg, milk and Parmesan in a shallow bowl. Add the bread and press it down lightly to immerse it in the egg mixture.

2. Heat the butter in a nonstick frying pan over a medium heat. Add the egg-soaked bread and cook for 2–3 minutes on each side until golden and slightly crisp. Cut into fingers and serve.

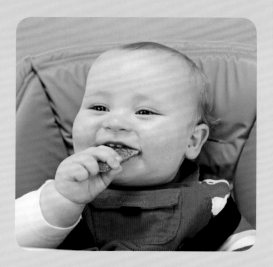

Our friends say...

'It was a revelation when my health visitor told me that babies don't need teeth to eat finger foods! They can manage certain soft foods really well by mashing them between their gums as the gums harden.'

Apple + sardine soldiers

serves 4 | prep 10 minutes | cook 10 minutes

Sardines are a fantastic source of healthy fats for your little soldier and make a brilliant store-cupboard ingredient for when you're short of time.

What you need

1 **eating apple**, peeled, cored and diced

40 g/1½ oz canned **sardines** in water, drained and bones removed

1 tablespoon **lemon juice**

1 teaspoon **paprika**

Toast or **pitta bread**, cut into fingers, to serve

What to do

1. Place the apple and 1 tablespoon of water in a small saucepan, cover with a lid and simmer over a low heat for 8 minutes until very soft. Using the back of a fork, mash the apple until smooth.

2. Meanwhile, mash the sardines and lemon juice in a bowl until smooth. Stir in the puréed apple and paprika and mix together until combined. Serve thinly spread on toast fingers or in a bowl for dunking the toast into.

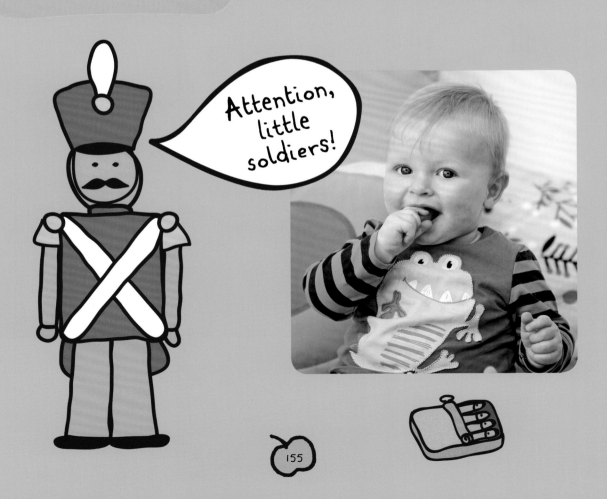

Attention, little soldiers!

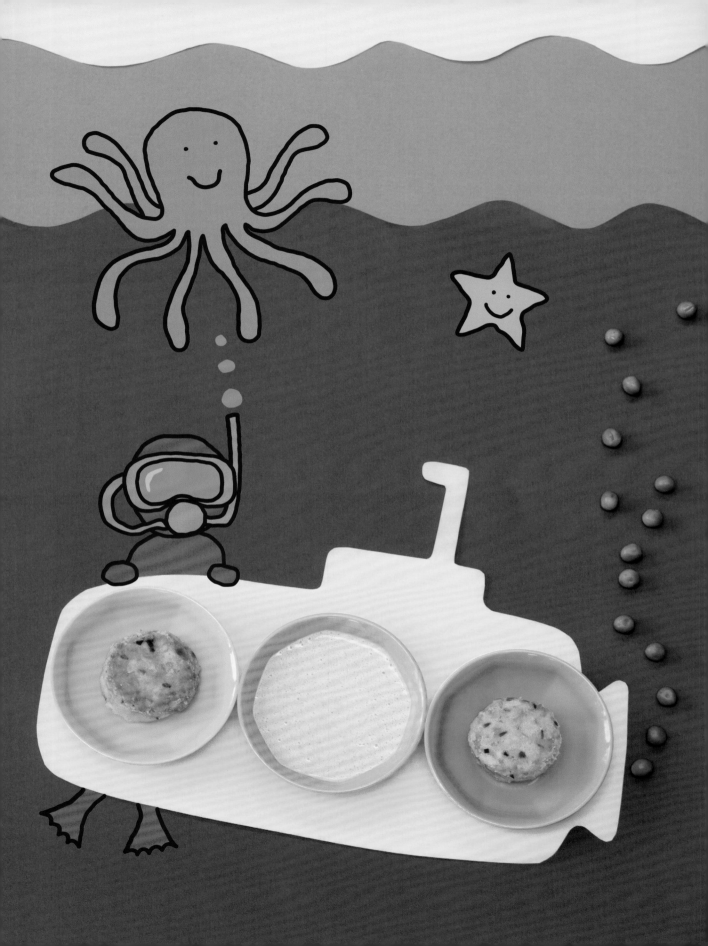

Squishy tuna fishcakes + mushy pea dip

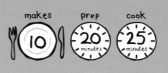

makes 10 · prep 20 minutes · cook 25 minutes

Dips at teatime are such fun and these tasty little fishcakes are perfect for dunking! They are yummy on their own, or try them with some green veg and rice if your little one is very hungry.

What you need

280 g/10 oz **potatoes**, halved

1 small **carrot**, peeled and chopped

60 g/2¼ oz canned **tuna chunks** in spring water, drained

1 tablespoon very finely snipped **chives**

1 teaspoon **Dijon mustard**

15 g/½ oz **unsalted butter**, melted

3 tablespoons **plain flour**, plus extra for dusting

2 tablespoons **olive oil**

For the mushy pea dip

175 g/6 oz **frozen peas**

2 tablespoons **thick natural yogurt**

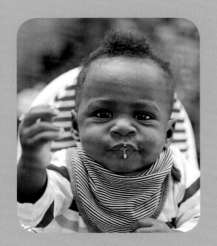

What to do

1. Cook the potatoes in boiling water for 12–15 minutes until tender, adding the carrot for the last 7 minutes of cooking time.

2. Meanwhile, make the mushy pea dip. Cook the peas in boiling water for 3 minutes until tender. Drain, reserving the cooking water. Purée the peas with 5 tablespoons of the reserved water in a food processor, or using a hand blender, until the peas are broken down and the mixture is smooth. To make the purée smoother, pass it through a sieve after blending. Mix the pea purée with the yogurt to combine. Transfer to a bowl and set aside.

3. Drain the potatoes and leave to dry and cool slightly, then peel off the skins and coarsely grate into a large bowl. Using the back of a fork, mash the carrot until almost smooth. Mash the tuna and add to the bowl with the potatoes. Add the carrot, chives, mustard and melted butter, then stir well.

4. Place the flour in a shallow bowl and dust your hands with a little extra flour. Divide the potato mixture into 10 equal pieces and shape into 10 patties. Lightly dust each patty in flour until coated all over.

5. Heat the oil in a large, nonstick frying pan over a medium heat and cook the tuna fishcakes for 3 minutes on each side until golden. Drain on kitchen paper. Serve with the mushy pea dip.

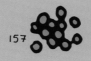

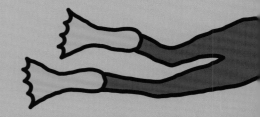

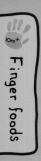
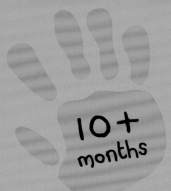

10+ months

By 10 months little foodies will have started to master their pincer grip so that they can pick up smaller pieces of food, such as strips of meat.

Pick-up porridge bars

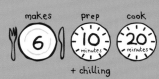

makes **6** | prep **10** minutes | cook **20** minutes

+ chilling

Sometimes busy babies need an extra breakfast boost when they head out on a morning adventure. These porridge bars are perfect at home or on the road.

What you need

40 g/1½ oz **porridge oats**

220 ml/7½ fl oz **whole milk**

20 g/¾ oz **raisins**, finely chopped

1 teaspoon **ground cinnamon**

10 g/¼ oz **unsalted butter**

What to do

1. Line a small baking tray with baking parchment. Place the oats and milk in a small saucepan and bring to the boil, then reduce the heat and simmer for 10 minutes, stirring frequently, or until the oats are soft.

2. Transfer to a bowl and stir in the raisins and cinnamon, then spread out the porridge in the tray to about 1 cm/½ inch thick. Cover with clingfilm and chill for 30 minutes to set.

3. Cut the porridge into 6 fingers each 7 cm/ 2¾ inches long by 2.5 cm/1 inch wide. Melt the butter in a nonstick frying pan and cook the fingers for 2–3 minutes on each side until golden.

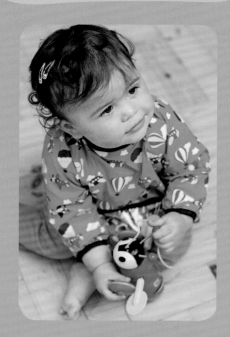

Really raisin-y soda bread

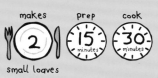
makes **2** small loaves · prep **15** minutes · cook **30** minutes

Soda bread is the easiest bread of all to make – just knead everything together and pop it in the oven! Slices from these little loaves are perfect for an energy boost at snacktimes.

What you need

355 g/12½ oz **plain wholemeal flour**, plus extra for dusting

1 teaspoon **bicarbonate of soda**

2 teaspoons **ground mixed spice**

125 g/4½ oz **raisins**, finely chopped

185 ml/6½ fl oz **buttermilk**

1 large **egg**, lightly beaten

What to do

1. Preheat the oven to 200°C/400°F/Gas Mark 6. Dust a baking sheet with flour.

2. Sift the flour into a large bowl, adding any bran left in the sieve. Stir in the bicarbonate of soda, mixed spice and raisins.

3. Whisk together the buttermilk and egg in a jug, then stir into the dry ingredients. Using a fork and then your hands, mix together to make a dough. Tip the dough onto a floured work surface, divide into 2 pieces and knead each to form into round loaves.

4. Place the loaves on the baking sheet, sprinkle over a little flour and make a cross-shaped cut halfway into the loaves. Bake for 30 minutes, or until risen and golden. Cool on a wire rack.

Can I help?

Knead it together

Sit your baby in a high chair at a table and when you come to the kneading part of the method, take your little one's hands in yours to work the dough together. Squishy and springy all at once!

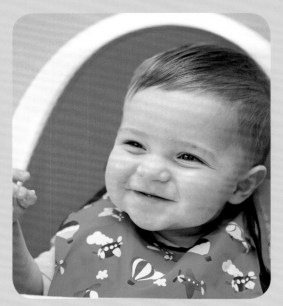

Ruby red mini-muffins

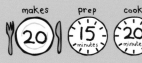

makes **20** | prep **15** minutes | cook **20** minutes

The bright colour of these muffins makes them irresistible to little hands. Best of all, the sweetness comes from beetroot and carrot, so there's no need for any naughty ingredients!

What you need

55 g/2 oz **unsalted butter**, melted, plus extra for greasing

140 g/5 oz **plain flour**

¼ teaspoon **bicarbonate of soda**

1 teaspoon **baking powder**

1 large **egg**, lightly beaten

150 ml/¼ pint **natural yogurt**

30 g/1 oz **feta cheese**, grated

1 small **carrot**, peeled and grated

100 g/3½ oz **cooked beetroot** (not in vinegar), patted dry and grated

1 tablespoon finely chopped **thyme** leaves

What to do

1. Preheat the oven to 190°C/375°F/Gas Mark 5. Grease 20 holes of 1 or 2 mini-muffin tins.

2. Sift the flour, bicarbonate of soda and baking powder into a large bowl and stir until combined, then make a well in the centre.

3. Beat together the egg, yogurt and melted butter in a bowl, then gradually pour into the dry ingredients and add the feta, carrot, beetroot and thyme. Using a wooden spoon, stir together gently but thoroughly until just combined.

4. Divide the mixture evenly among the prepared muffin holes, then bake in the oven for 15–20 minutes until risen. Leave to cool slightly, then cool completely on a wire rack.

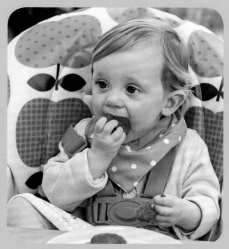

Our friends say...

'Finger foods saved me with baby number two! They meant I could give the little one something to hold and munch on while I fed the older one. Then, I could come back to the baby to complete his meal with a purée.'

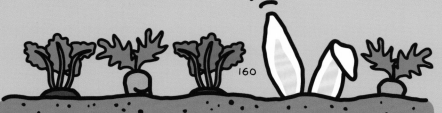

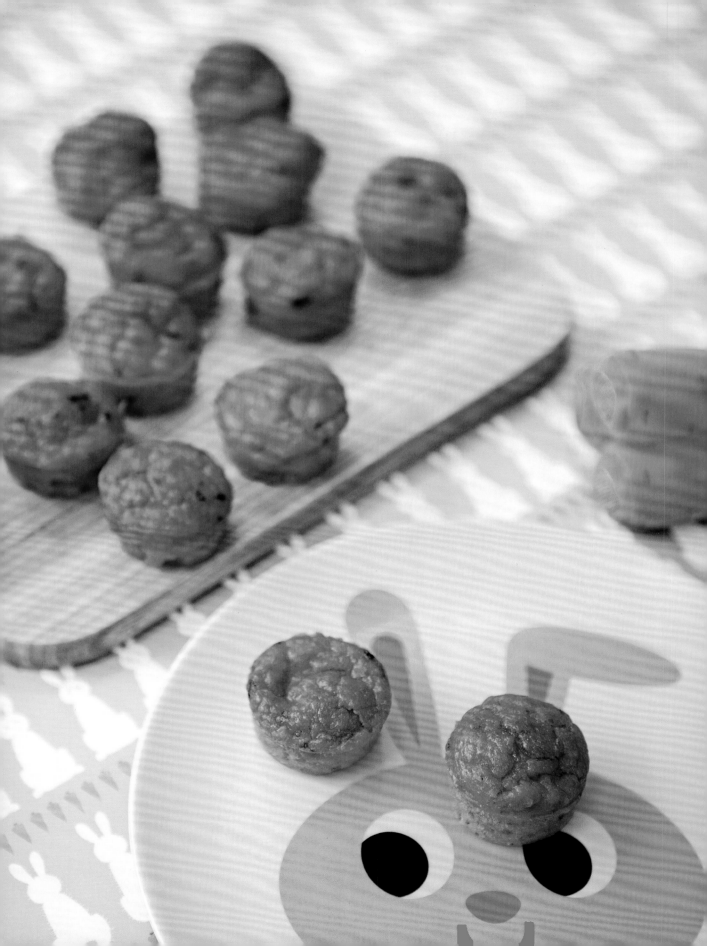

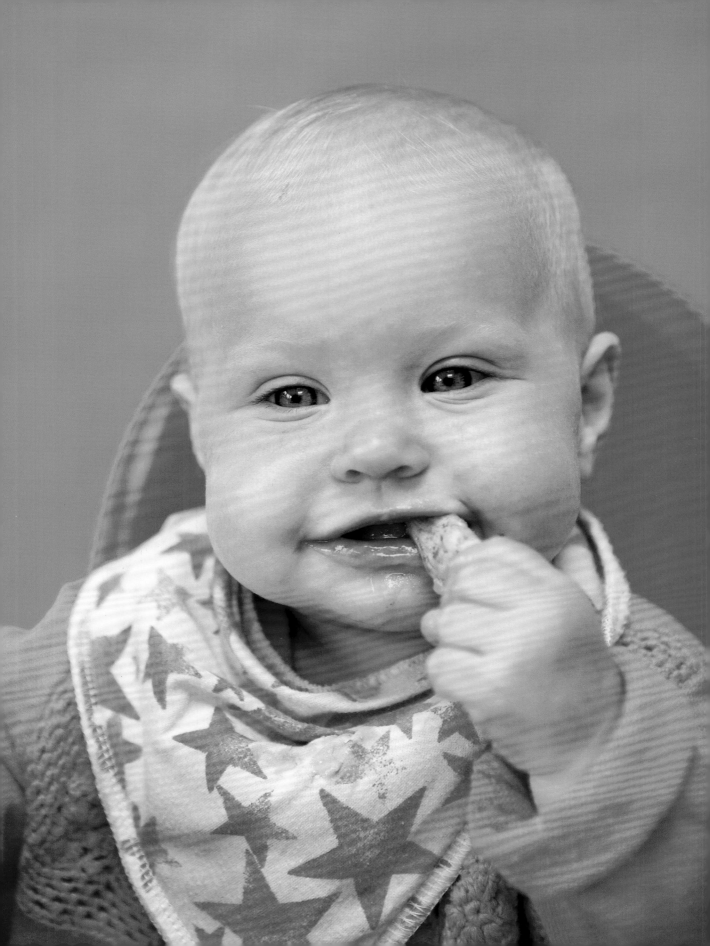

Dunk-me satay chicken

Your baby will love dunking these juicy strips of chicken in the golden peanutty sauce. They are also perfect served cold for a picnic.

What you need

1 teaspoon **smoked paprika**

1 tablespoon **olive oil**

1 skinless **chicken breast** (about 150 g/5½ oz), cut into 4–6 strips

Steamed **carrot sticks** and **mangetout**, to serve

For the satay sauce

3 tablespoons no-salt, no-sugar **smooth peanut butter**

½ teaspoon reduced-salt **soy sauce**

2 tablespoons **coconut milk** or **mayonnaise**

What to do

1. Mix together the paprika and 1 teaspoon of the olive oil in a shallow dish and add the chicken. Stir until the chicken is coated and leave to marinate while you make the satay sauce.

2. Mix together the peanut butter, soy sauce, coconut milk or mayonnaise and 1–2 tablespoons of warm water in a small bowl until combined. Set aside.

3. Heat the remaining oil in a nonstick frying pan over a medium–high heat and cook the chicken for 2–3 minutes on each side until golden and cooked through. Serve the chicken with the satay sauce and carrot and mangetout.

Feed the senses

Crumbly coconut dough

We think using food for play is one of the best ways to make sure children have lots of happy thoughts about the things they eat. Try making this special play dough – it smells good enough to eat and it's really crumbly! All you have to do is mix one part coconut milk with two parts cornflour. Give it a good stir (ask your little one for help) to combine, then push it together with your hands. The more you play, the crumblier it gets, but that yummy smell keeps on going!

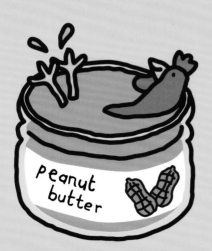

peanut butter

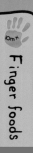

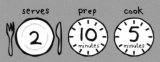

serves 2 · prep 10 minutes · cook 5 minutes

Dippy pea guacamole

Chunks of avocado can be very slippery to hold onto, so to make it easier try mashing them up with some peas – perfect for dipping veggie sticks in.

What you need

30 g/1 oz **frozen petits pois**

½ small **avocado**, stoned

1 teaspoon **lime or lemon juice**

3 tablespoons **baby's usual milk**

A few **coriander** leaves, finely chopped (optional)

1 soft **wholemeal tortilla**, cut into fingers, to serve

Steamed **vegetable sticks**, to serve

What to do

1. Steam or boil the petits pois in a small saucepan over a medium heat for 3–4 minutes until tender. Drain, if necessary, and tip into a bowl.

2. Scoop out the avocado flesh into the bowl and pour in the citrus juice and milk. Using the back of a fork, mash together until almost smooth. Alternatively, purée using a hand blender. To make the purée smoother, pass it through a sieve after blending.

3. Stir in the coriander (if using). Serve with the tortilla and vegetable sticks.

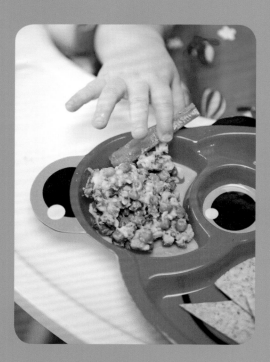

Our friends say...

'Some slippery foods, such as banana or avocado, were really tricky for my little one to pick up. So, I would coat the pieces in wheatgerm (which is nutritious, too!) to make them easier for his little hands to grasp hold of.'

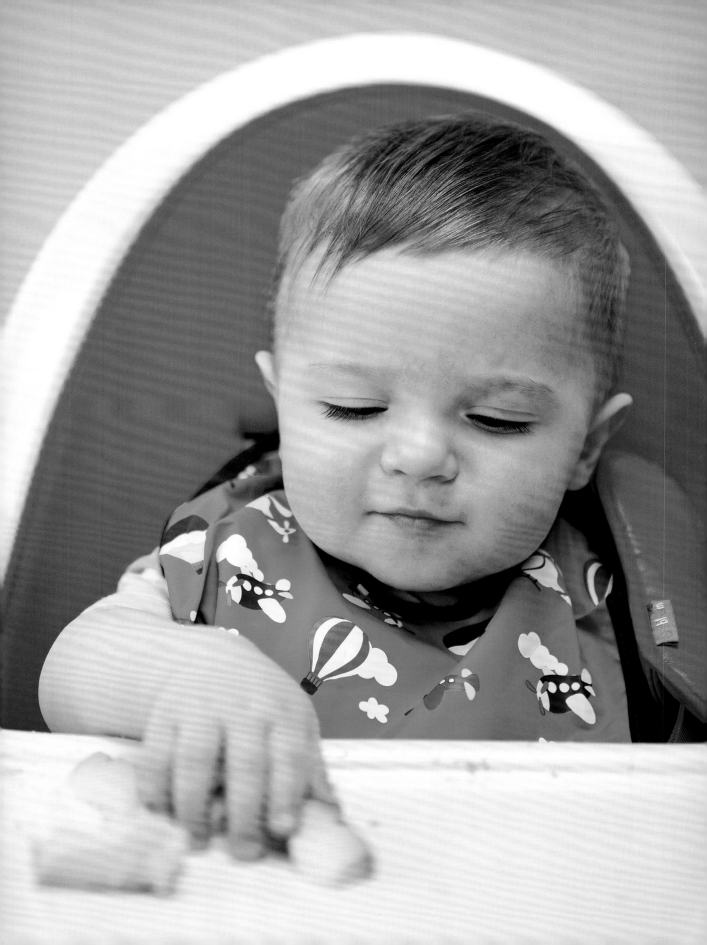

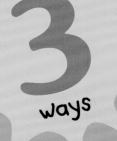
3 ways

Three ways with heavenly hummus

Here are 3 of our favourite ways to add some va-va-voom to the creamy, nutty taste of hummus. Serve with veggie sticks or toasted pitta fingers.

Really red hummus

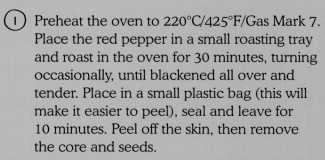

makes 10 portions — prep 20 minutes — cook 30 minutes

What you need

1 **red pepper**

120 g/4¼ oz canned **chickpeas** in water, drained

4 teaspoons **lemon juice**

2 tablespoons **light tahini**

1 small **garlic** clove, finely chopped

1 tablespoon **extra virgin olive oil**

What to do

1. Preheat the oven to 220°C/425°F/Gas Mark 7. Place the red pepper in a small roasting tray and roast in the oven for 30 minutes, turning occasionally, until blackened all over and tender. Place in a small plastic bag (this will make it easier to peel), seal and leave for 10 minutes. Peel off the skin, then remove the core and seeds.

2. Place the pepper flesh with any juices in a food processor or blender, add the chickpeas, lemon, tahini, garlic, oil and 2 tablespoons of water and whiz until smooth and creamy.

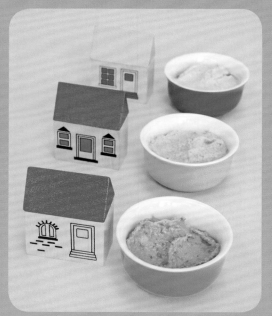

Our friends say...

'Introduce finger foods as soon as you can. I didn't give my first baby any until he was over 11 months and it took him ages to get the hang of feeding himself. For my second, I introduced them around 7 months, and she was much quicker.'

Brilliant butternut hummus

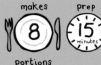

makes **8** portions · prep **15** minutes · cook **15** minutes

What you need

125 g/4½ oz **butternut squash**, peeled, deseeded and cubed

120 g/4¼ oz canned **chickpeas** in water, drained

2 tablespoons **lemon juice**

2 tablespoons **light tahini**

1 small **garlic** clove, finely chopped

1 tablespoon **extra virgin olive oil**

½ teaspoon **ground cumin**

What to do

1. Steam or boil the butternut squash in a saucepan over a medium heat for 10–15 minutes until tender.

2. Transfer the squash to a food processor or blender, add the chickpeas, lemon juice, tahini, garlic, oil, cumin and 2 tablespoons of water and whiz until smooth and creamy.

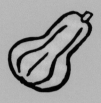

Nice + nutty hummus

makes **6** portions · prep **10** minutes · cook **no cook**

What you need

120 g/4¼ oz canned **chickpeas** in water, drained

2 tablespoons **lemon juice**

1 tablespoon **light tahini**

1 tablespoon no-salt, no-sugar **smooth peanut butter**

1 small **garlic** clove, finely chopped

1 tablespoon **extra virgin olive oil**

½ teaspoon **ground cumin**

What to do

1. Place the chickpeas, lemon juice, tahini, peanut butter, garlic, oil, cumin and 2 tablespoons of water in a food processor or blender and whiz until smooth and creamy.

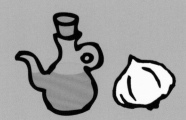

Dinky courgette fritters

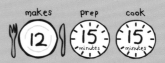

makes 12 • prep 15 minutes • cook 15 minutes

Fresh mint makes these courgette fritters especially tasty. Tiny fingers will love exploring the crispy texture, too!

What you need

1 **courgette**, coarsely grated

30 g/1 oz **plain flour**

1 **egg**, lightly beaten

3 tablespoons finely grated **Parmesan cheese**

2 tablespoons very finely chopped **mint** leaves (optional)

Olive oil, for frying

What to do

1. Squeeze the grated courgette in a clean tea towel to remove any excess water, then tip it into a large bowl. Stir in the flour, egg, Parmesan and mint (if using) to make a loose batter.

2. Heat enough oil to coat the base of a large, nonstick frying pan over a medium heat. Add 1 heaped tablespoon of the courgette mixture per fritter and cook in 2 batches for 2–3 minutes on each side until golden. Drain on kitchen paper before serving.

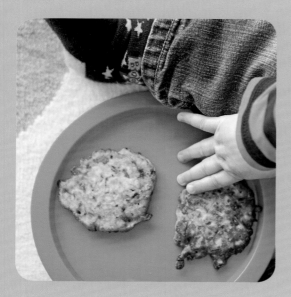

Our friends say...

'I love thinking of fun ways to use food for play. One of my baby's favourites is when I use a whole courgette as a microphone. Sometimes I make him giggle by singing into it; and sometimes I use it to "interview" him about how much he loves what he's eating!'

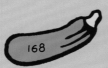

Crunchy munchy polenta fish fingers

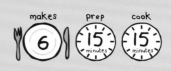
makes **6** | prep **15** minutes | cook **15** minutes

Fish fingers were made for eating with little hands – it's in the name! These are made with polenta for extra-special crunchiness and a little lemon for a citrus tang.

What you need

2 teaspoons **olive oil**

2 tablespoons **plain flour**

1 **egg**, lightly beaten

4 tablespoons **instant polenta**

Finely grated rind of ½ **lemon**

2 skinless, boneless **cod or salmon fillets** or other firm fish (about 115 g/4 oz each), cut widthways into 2.5 cm/ 1 inch-wide fingers

What to do

1. Preheat the oven to 190°C/375°F/Gas Mark 5. Brush the oil over a large baking sheet.

2. Place the flour in a shallow dish and the beaten egg in a bowl. Place the polenta into a second shallow dish and mix in the lemon rind. Dip each fish finger into the flour, then the egg, followed by the polenta, and place on the prepared baking sheet.

3. Bake the fish fingers in the preheated oven for 10–15 minutes, turning the fish over halfway through the cooking time, until golden and cooked through. Serve with your little one's favourite veggies.

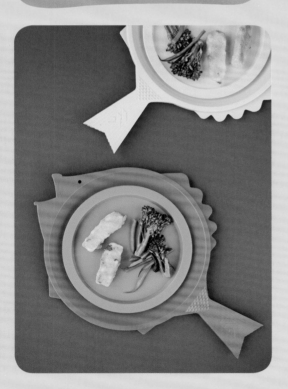

Just for fun

Polenta pictures

The grainy texture of polenta makes it perfect for drawing pictures. Pour some polenta onto a tray (a dark-coloured tray works best) and show your little one how to use a finger to draw simple pictures in the grains.

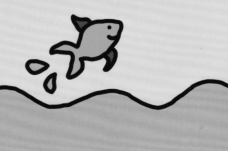

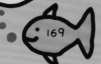

Slurpy smoothie lollies

 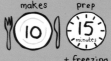
What you need

1 large **mango** (about 650 g/
   1 lb 7 oz), peeled, stoned
   and chopped

1 **banana** (about 150 g/5½ oz),
   roughly chopped

200 g/7 oz **fresh or frozen
   raspberries**

200 ml/7 fl oz **whole milk**

1 teaspoon **vanilla extract**

What to do

① Place the mango, banana, raspberries, milk
   and vanilla extract in a food processor or
   blender and blend until smooth and creamy.

② Pour the fruit mixture into 10 small lolly
   moulds (shapes are especially good fun)
   and freeze for 3 hours until frozen solid.

Chomp-chomp cookies

 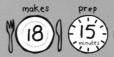

What you need

30 g/1 oz **dried cherries**,
   finely chopped

100 g/3½ oz **porridge oats**

50 g/1¾ oz **ground almonds**

100 g/3½ oz **desiccated
   unsweetened coconut**

½ teaspoon **ground cinnamon**

½ teaspoon **baking powder**

2 large ripe **bananas**, peeled

½ teaspoon **vanilla extract**

5 tablespoons **olive oil**

What to do

① Preheat the oven to 180°C/350°F/Gas Mark 4.
   Line 2 baking sheets with baking parchment.

② Mix together the chopped cherries, oats,
   ground almonds, desiccated coconut,
   cinnamon and baking powder in a large bowl.

③ In a second bowl, mash the bananas, then
   stir in the vanilla extract and oil. Combine
   the wet and dry ingredients.

④ Place heaped tablespoons of the mixture onto
   the prepared baking sheets, then flatten the
   tops slightly to make cookies about 3.5 cm/
   1½ inches in diameter. Bake in the oven for
   15–20 minutes until golden and slightly crisp.
   Leave to cool on the sheets for a few minutes,
   then cool completely on a wire rack.

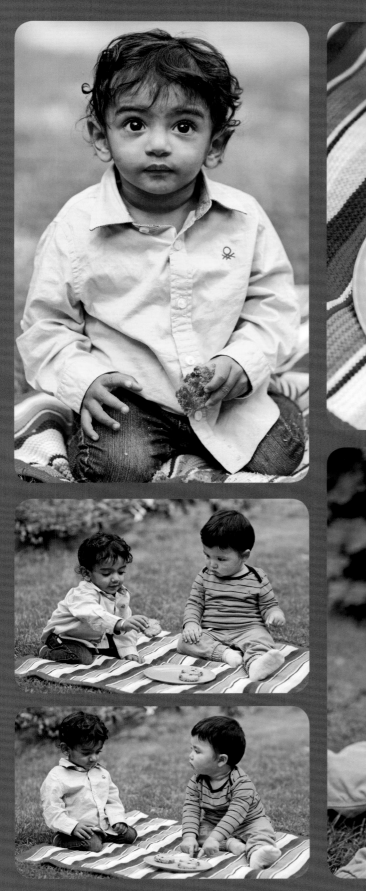

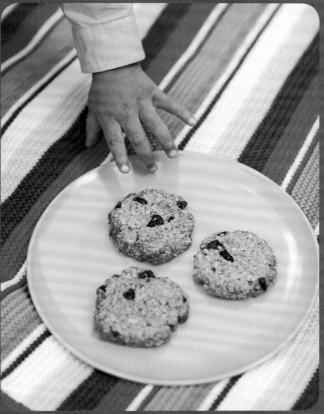

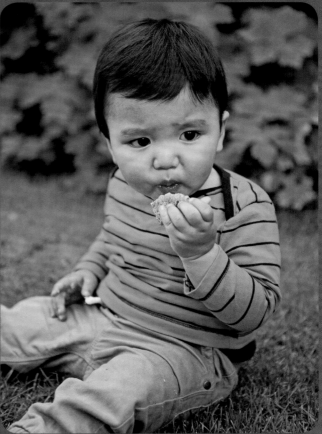

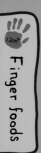

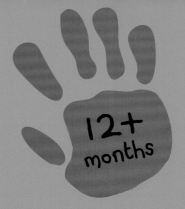

12+ months

By 12 months little ones can be really good at holding food and using their chompy teeth for biting. Now they can really enjoy feeding themselves!

Crispy veggie fingers

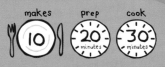

makes 10 | prep 20 minutes | cook 30 minutes

Crispy and creamy, with a hint of a mustard twist, these fingers are made with heaps of veg – and are a brilliant way to make use of veggie leftovers after a Sunday roast.

What you need

325 g/11½ oz **potatoes**, halved

55 g/2 oz **green cabbage**, chopped

90 g/3¼ oz **frozen petits pois**

3 **spring onions**, finely chopped

1 teaspoon **English mustard powder**

4 tablespoons **cottage cheese**

1 **egg**, lightly beaten

85 g/3 oz **fresh breadcrumbs**

Sunflower oil, for frying

What to do

1. Cook the potatoes in a saucepan of boiling water for 12–15 minutes until tender. Drain and leave to dry and cool slightly, then peel off the skins and coarsely grate into a large bowl.

2. Meanwhile, steam or boil the cabbage and petits pois over a medium heat for 3–4 minutes until tender, then finely chop. Add to the potatoes with the spring onions, mustard and cottage cheese. Mix until combined.

3. Place the beaten egg in a bowl and the breadcrumbs on a plate. Divide the potato mixture into 10 equal pieces and shape into croquettes. Dip each croquette into the beaten egg, then roll in the breadcrumbs until each one is coated all over.

4. Heat enough oil to generously cover the base of a large, nonstick frying pan and cook the croquettes in 2 batches over a medium heat for 5–7 minutes, turning occasionally, until golden all over.

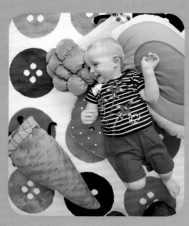

Crumbly creamy salmon parcels

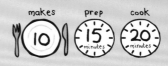

makes 10 | prep 15 minutes | cook 20 minutes

What you need

Unsalted butter, for greasing

165 g/5¾ oz (about ½ pack) **ready-rolled puff pastry**, cut in half lengthways

Plain flour, for dusting

2 skinless, boneless **salmon fillets** (about 115 g/4 oz each), cut into 1 cm/½ inch cubes

A small handful of **dill**, finely chopped

3 tablespoons **cream cheese**

1 teaspoon **lemon juice**

Beaten **egg**, to glaze

What to do

1. 1. Preheat the oven to 190°C/375°F/ Gas Mark 5. Lightly grease a baking sheet. Lay one piece of the pastry widthways on a floured surface and roll it to make it 2 cm/ ¾ inch wider.

2. Place the salmon in a bowl and combine with the dill, cream cheese and lemon juice.

3. Spoon half the mixture along the centre of the pastry. Brush a little beaten egg along one long edge of the pastry, then draw both edges over the filling; press to seal. Trim the edge. Repeat with the remaining pastry and filling.

4. Turn the pastry rolls seam-side down and cut into 10 equal pieces. Brush each one with beaten egg and place on the prepared baking sheet. Bake for 15–20 minutes until golden and cooked through.

Ham + egg bakies

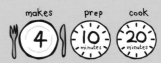

makes 4 | prep 10 minutes | cook 20 minutes

What you need

Olive oil, for greasing

4 thin round slices of **ham** (15 g/½ oz each)

4 **eggs**

2 **tomatoes**, deseeded and diced (optional)

Mashed potato and steamed **vegetable sticks**, to serve

What to do

1. Preheat the oven to 180°C/350°F/Gas Mark 4. Lightly grease 4 holes of a deep muffin tin.

2. Line the prepared muffin holes with the slices of ham. Crack an egg into each one and scatter the tomatoes (if using) over the top.

3. Bake in the oven for 18–20 minutes until the egg is set. Transfer to a wire rack and leave to cool slightly. Serve the pies with mashed potato and steamed vegetable sticks.

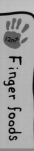

Terrific tortilla parcels

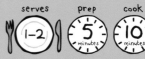

serves 1–2 prep 5 minutes cook 10 minutes

These tasty tortilla parcels are the ultimate in cheese on toast. The stringiness of the creamy mozzarella is super-oozy, making the parcels too delicious to resist!

What you need

1 small low-salt soft **tortilla**

2 slices of **mozzarella cheese** (about 30 g/1 oz total weight)

3 slices of **tomato**

A large pinch of **dried oregano**

Olive oil, for brushing

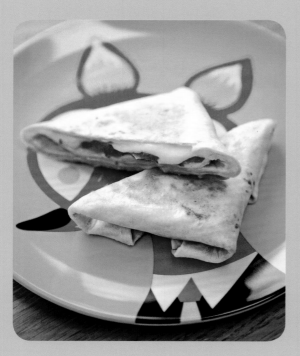

What to do

1. Place the tortilla in a dry, nonstick frying pan over a medium heat and warm slightly to make it easier to fold.

2. Lay the mozzarella and tomato in the centre of the warm tortilla, then sprinkle the oregano over the top. Fold in the sides to make a square parcel and enclose the filling.

3. Brush the tortilla all over with a little oil and cook in the frying pan, seam side down, for 2–3 minutes, then turn it over and cook for a further 2–3 minutes until golden and starting to crisp. Remove from the heat, cool for a few minutes, then cut diagonally in half.

Add some zing!

For an added zing in your little one's tortilla parcels, spread a thin layer of homemade red pesto (see p.54) over the inside of the tortilla before you fill and wrap it.

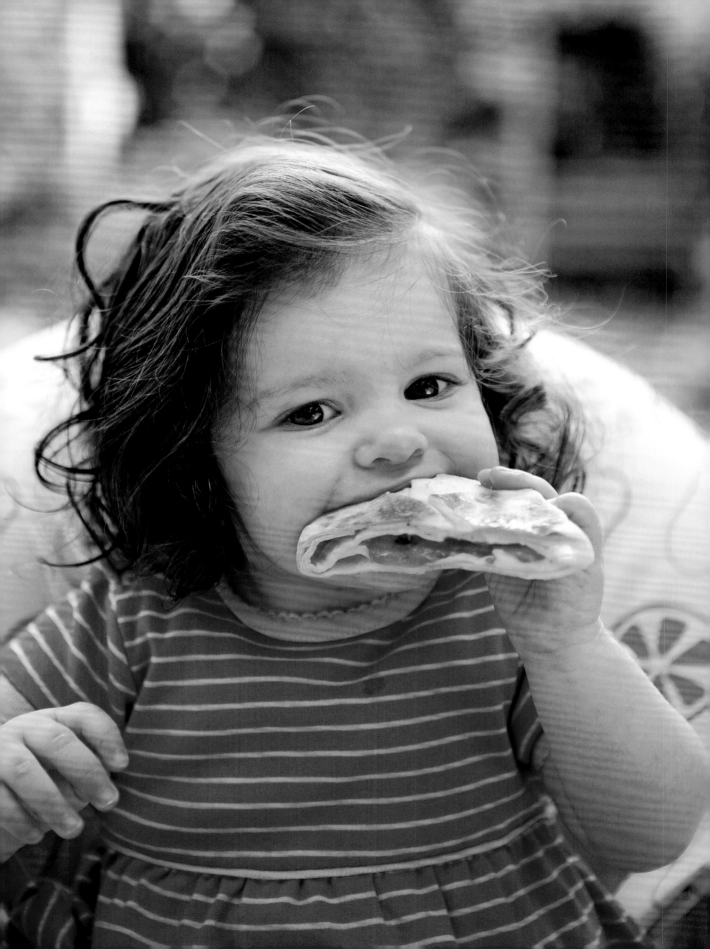

Round + round rice bites

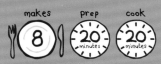

makes **8** | prep **20** minutes | cook **20** minutes

The crispy edge, oozy middle and soft rice make these rice bites an explosion of textures on your little one's tongue – and they are such a great way to use up leftover risotto.

What you need

Olive oil, for greasing and drizzling

165 g/5¾ oz **cooked risotto rice** (see p.89, or make fresh using just rice and stock)

1 **egg**, lightly beaten

30 g/1 oz **fresh breadcrumbs**

15 g/½ oz **mozzarella cheese**, cut into 8 cubes

1 slice of **Parma ham**, finely chopped

What to do

1. Preheat the oven to 220°C/425°F/Gas Mark 7. Lightly grease a baking sheet.

2. Place the risotto in a bowl, mash lightly with the back of a fork and stir in the egg to make a loose paste. Place the breadcrumbs in a separate bowl.

3. Using wet hands, shape a walnut-sized piece of the rice mixture into a ball, then press a cube of mozzarella into the centre, sprinkle over the finely chopped ham and form the rice around the filling to enclose. The mixture is quite loose but will hold together when cooked. Dip the ball into the breadcrumbs until coated all over, then transfer to the prepared baking sheet. Repeat with the remaining rice and fillings to make 8 walnut-sized balls.

4. Drizzle a little oil over each rice ball, then bake in the oven for 15–20 minutes, turning once, until golden all over and the rice is piping hot inside. Leave to cool slightly before serving.

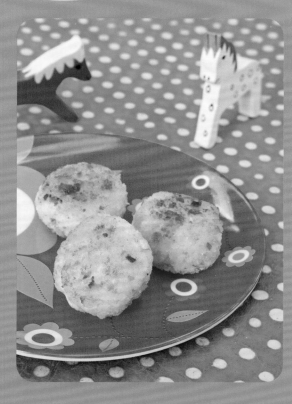

Can I help?

Take a dip!

Older little ones might like to have a go at dipping the rice balls in the breadcrumbs. Careful not to squish them!

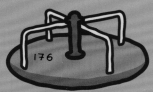

Big + strong muffins

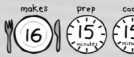

Crammed with spinach, cheese and a little bit of mustard, these muffins not only pack a big, tasty punch they also have iron for making strong little immune systems.

What you need

50 g/1¾ oz **unsalted butter**, melted, plus extra for greasing

150 g/5½ oz **self-raising flour**

1 teaspoon **baking powder**

1 teaspoon **English mustard powder**

50 g/1¾ oz **baby spinach leaves**, stalks removed and leaves very finely chopped

100 g/3½ oz no-salt, no-sugar canned **sweetcorn**, drained

30 g/1 oz **mature Cheddar cheese**, finely grated

125 ml/4 fl oz **whole milk**

1 **egg**, lightly beaten

What to do

1. Preheat the oven to 190°C/375°F/Gas Mark 5. Grease 16 holes of 1 or 2 mini-muffin tins.

2. Sift the flour, baking powder and mustard powder into a large bowl. Stir in the spinach, sweetcorn and the cheese until fully combined, then make a well in the centre.

3. Beat together the milk, egg and melted butter in a jug, then gradually pour into the dry ingredients and gently stir together with a wooden spoon until just combined.

4. Divide the mixture evenly among the prepared muffin holes, then bake the muffins in the oven for 12–15 minutes until risen and golden. Cool on a wire rack. Serve warm or cold.

Our friends say...

'I loved telling my little ones why their food was good for them – "Spinach makes you *reeeally* strong!" and "Milk and cheese give you superhero bones and gnashy teeth!" I think it's good for them to know that food isn't just about filling hungry tummies.'

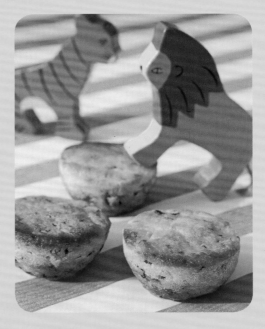

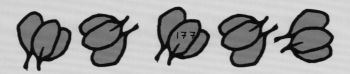

Rainbow veg + chicken kebabs

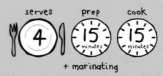

serves 4 | prep 15 minutes | cook 15 minutes
+ marinating

These tasty little sticks of flavoursome chicken and veggies are great fun for little ones to eat. Try using lots of different types of veg to find your baby's favourite combo.

What you need

1 tablespoon **olive oil**, plus extra for brushing

1 **garlic** clove, crushed

1 cm/½ inch piece of fresh **root ginger**, peeled and finely chopped

1 teaspoon **Chinese 5-spice**

1 teaspoon **clear honey**

2 large, skinless **chicken breasts** (about 175 g/6 oz each), cut into bite-sized chunks

1 **red pepper**, cored, deseeded and cut into bite-sized pieces

1 **courgette**, cut into bite-sized slices

What to do

1. Mix together the oil, garlic, ginger, 5-spice and honey in a shallow dish. Add the chicken pieces and turn until well coated. Cover with clingfilm and leave to marinate in the fridge for at least 15 minutes.

2. Preheat the grill to high and line the grill pan with aluminium foil. Remove the chicken from the marinade and thread onto 4 short skewers, alternating with the red pepper and courgette. Brush the chicken with any remaining marinade and brush the vegetables with a little oil.

3. Grill the kebabs for 10–15 minutes, turning frequently, until golden and cooked through. Take the chicken and vegetables off the skewers before serving, and chop into pincer-grip bite-sized chunks.

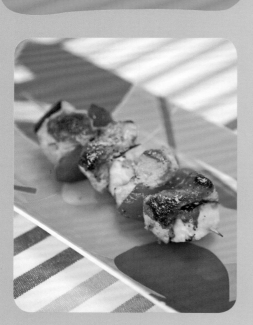

Gingerly gingery

Feed the senses

Fresh root ginger is fascinating for little hands to hold and explore – look at all those knobbly bits, like the bark on a tree! Give a piece to your baby to hold, and cut off one end so that you can both have a good sniff, too – *reeeally* smelly!

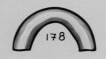

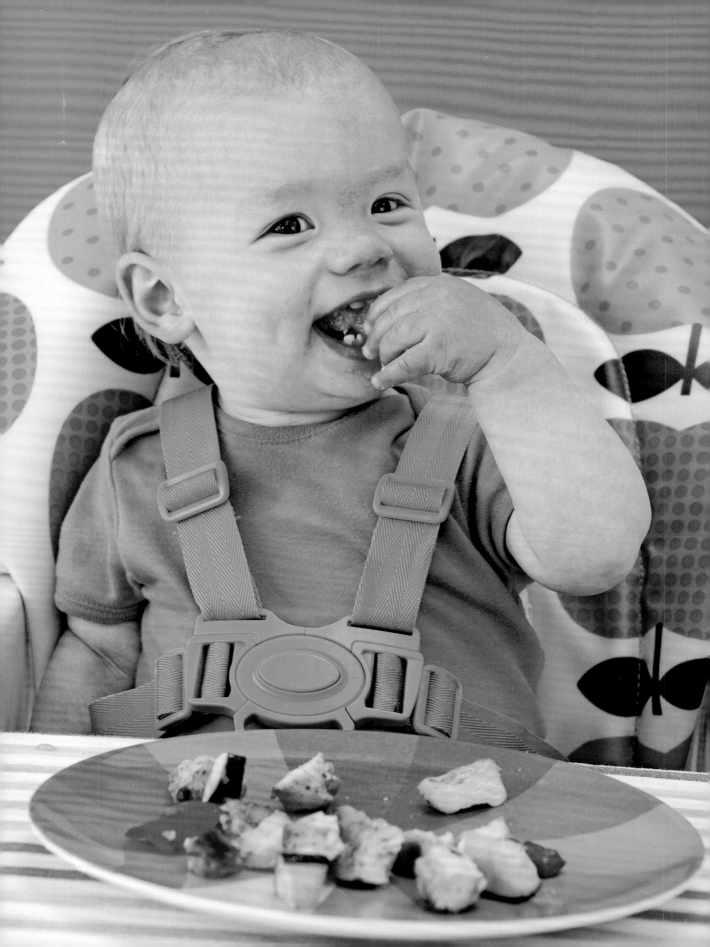

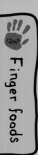
Mighty fine falafels with mega-minty dip

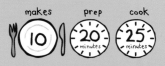

makes **10** · prep **20** minutes · cook **25** minutes

Chickpeas are a brilliant source of protein for growing explorers. Warming spices make these patties really tasty. They're especially yummy dunked in the minty dip.

What you need

2 tablespoons **olive oil**, plus extra if needed

1 **onion**, finely chopped

1 **garlic** clove, crushed

1 teaspoon **ground cumin**

1 teaspoon **ground coriander**

400 g/14 oz can **chickpeas** in water, drained and rinsed

6 unsulphured, dark **dried apricots**, finely chopped

A large handful of **coriander** leaves, finely chopped

1 **egg**, lightly beaten

3 tablespoons **plain flour**, plus extra for dusting

Small **pitta breads**, to serve

For the mega-minty dip

6 tablespoons **natural yogurt**

2 tablespoons finely chopped **mint** leaves

What to do

1. To make the minty yogurt dip, mix together the yogurt and mint in a bowl. Set aside until ready to serve.

2. To make the falafels, heat half the oil in a large, nonstick frying pan over a medium heat and cook the onion for 5 minutes, stirring frequently, until softened. Reduce the heat to low, add the garlic, cumin and ground coriander and cook for 2 minutes, stirring.

3. Tip the onion mixture into a food processor, add the chickpeas and whiz until fairly smooth. Alternatively, transfer to a bowl and mash with a potato masher. Add the apricots, coriander leaves and egg and mix together until thoroughly combined.

4. Place the flour in a shallow bowl and dust your hands with a little extra flour. Divide the mixture into 10 equal pieces and shape each one into a small, slightly squashed round – like a small patty. Lightly dust each falafel in the flour until coated all over.

5. Heat the remaining oil in the cleaned frying pan. Cook the falafels, in batches if necessary, over a medium heat for 8–10 minutes, turning frequently until golden and cooked through. Add a little extra oil to the pan, if needed. Drain on kitchen paper, then serve with the yogurt dip and pitta breads.

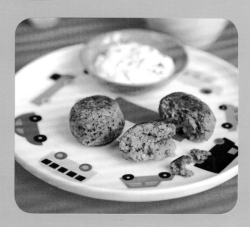

180

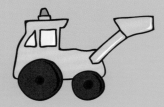

Banana + ricotta puffs

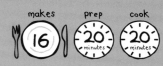

makes **16** | prep **20** minutes | cook **20** minutes

These little puffs of pure creaminess are *sooo* tempting. They are so easy to make that we recommend making a few extra so that grown-ups can nibble some, too!

What you need

Unsalted butter, for greasing

1 large ripe **banana**

2 tablespoons **ricotta cheese**

320 g/11¼ oz **ready-rolled puff pastry**

Plain flour, for dusting

Beaten **egg**, to glaze

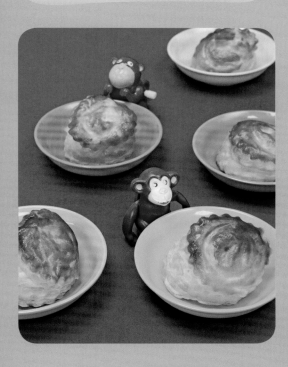

What to do

1. Preheat the oven to 200°C/400°F/Gas Mark 6. Lightly grease 2 baking sheets.

2. Using the back of a fork, roughly mash the banana in a bowl, then stir in the ricotta.

3. Lay the pastry on a lightly floured work surface and roll it out slightly. Stamp out rounds using a 5 cm/2 inch fluted cutter until you have 32 rounds (re-roll the trimmings as necessary). Place a heaped teaspoon of banana mixture in the centre of one round and brush the edge with beaten egg. Place a second pastry round on top and gently press the edges together to seal. Place the parcel on a prepared baking sheet and repeat with the remaining pastry and filling to make 16 parcels.

4. Lightly brush the top of each parcel with egg and prick with a fork. Bake for 18–20 minutes until risen and golden. Transfer to a wire rack to cool. Serve warm or cold.

Can I help?

Roll + press

With a little bit of grown-up help, your baby can have a go at rolling the pastry and pressing out the circles. Have fun squidging the leftover pastry pieces, too.

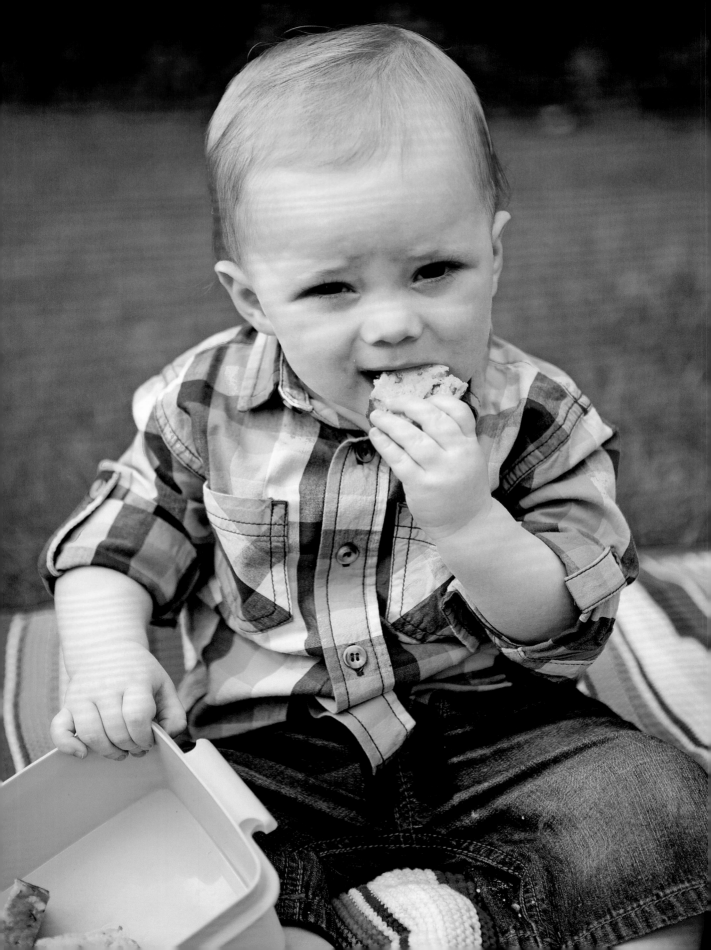

Hidden gems polenta loaf

makes **16** slices · prep **20** minutes · cook **35** minutes

Polenta gives this lovely loaf a special texture for little ones to explore, and the peppers give tiny flecks of colour to point to. Try this loaf served warm with a little butter. Yum!

What you need

60 g/2¼ oz **unsalted butter**, melted, plus extra for greasing

165 g/5¾ oz **instant polenta**

75 g/2½ oz **plain flour**

2 teaspoons **baking powder**

½ teaspoon **bicarbonate of soda**

2 teaspoons **English mustard powder**

1 **courgette**, grated

75 g/2½ oz **roasted peppers** from a jar, drained and finely chopped

50 g/1¾ oz **Cheddar cheese**, grated

2 large **eggs**, lightly beaten

185 ml/6½ fl oz **buttermilk**

50 ml/2 fl oz **whole milk**

What to do

1. Preheat the oven to 200°C/400°F/Gas Mark 6. Lightly grease a 450 g/1 lb loaf tin.

2. Mix together the polenta, flour, baking powder, bicarbonate of soda and mustard powder in a large bowl. Squeeze the courgette in a clean tea towel to remove any excess water and add to the dry ingredients with the peppers and cheese.

3. Beat together the eggs, melted butter, buttermilk and milk in a jug, then stir into the polenta mixture using a wooden spoon. Spoon into the prepared loaf tin and smooth the top.

4. Bake in the oven for 30–35 minutes until risen and a skewer inserted into the centre comes out clean. Leave to cool in the tin for 5 minutes, then turn out onto a wire rack and leave to cool completely before slicing.

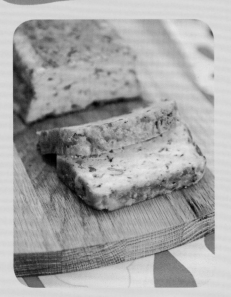

Our friends say...

'My baby was good at new flavours, but resistant to changes in texture. I didn't force him and didn't ever say "Don't you like it?" I just kept saying, "Let's try again tomorrow," so that, eventually, one day he'd have a go.'

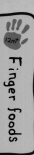

Super-seeds fridge bars

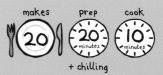

We love these bars because they are packed full of dried fruit, seeds and oats and you don't need to cook them. They are also lip-smackingly sticky! Once they're chilled, simply cut them into fingers and serve them as a tasty snack at home or on the go.

What you need

100 g/3½ oz **jumbo porridge oats**

25 g/1 oz **hazelnuts**

25 g/1 oz **blanched almonds**

3 tablespoons **sunflower seeds**

175 g/6 oz unsulphured, dark **dried apricots**, roughly chopped

75 g/2½ oz **raisins**

4 tablespoons **fresh orange juice**

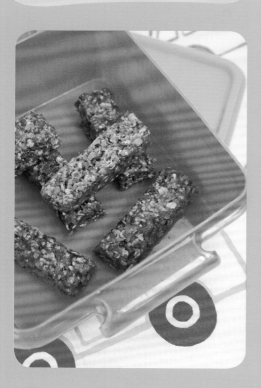

What to do

1. Line an 18-cm/7-inch square baking tin with baking parchment. Place the oats in a large, nonstick frying pan and dry-fry over a medium–low heat for 4–5 minutes, tossing frequently, until golden and crisp. Tip into a bowl and let cool.

2. Add the nuts to the pan and dry-fry over a medium–low heat for 2 minutes, then add the sunflower seeds and cook for a further 2 minutes, turning frequently, until golden. Tip into a separate bowl and allow to cool.

3. Place the apricots, raisins and orange juice in a food processor or blender and blend to a smooth, thick purée. Scrape the fruit into a large bowl.

4. Whiz the oats in the food processor or blender until coarsely chopped, then add them to the fruit purée. Finally, whiz the nuts and seeds until coarsely chopped and add to the bowl. Stir well until everything is combined.

5. Spread the fruit mixture in an even layer, about 1.5 cm/¾ inch thick, in the prepared tin. Chill for 1 hour until firm. Cut into 20 bars.

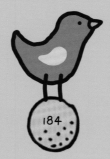

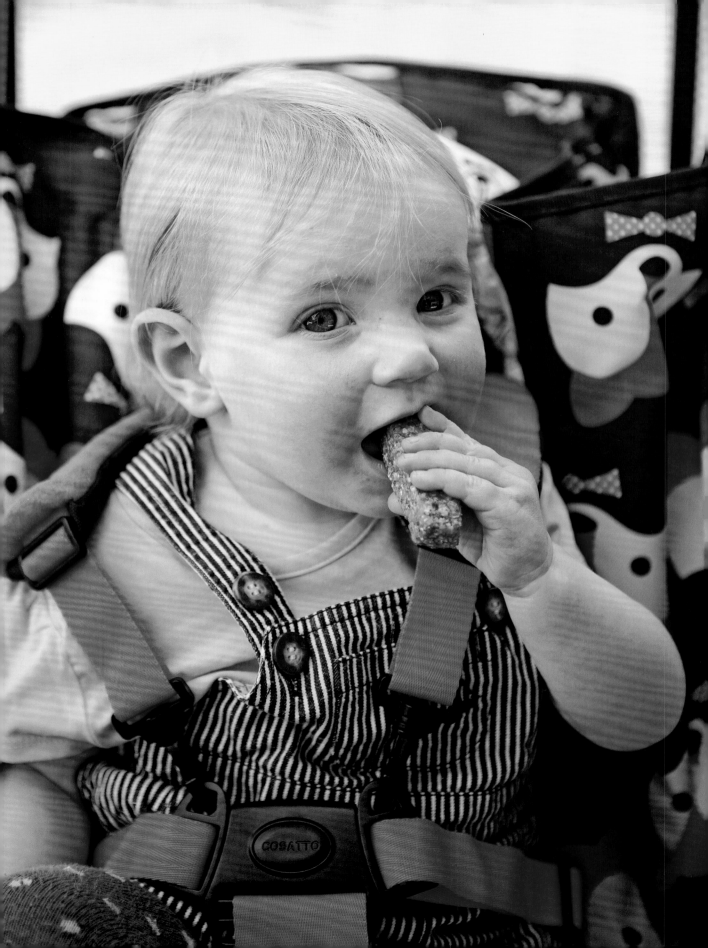

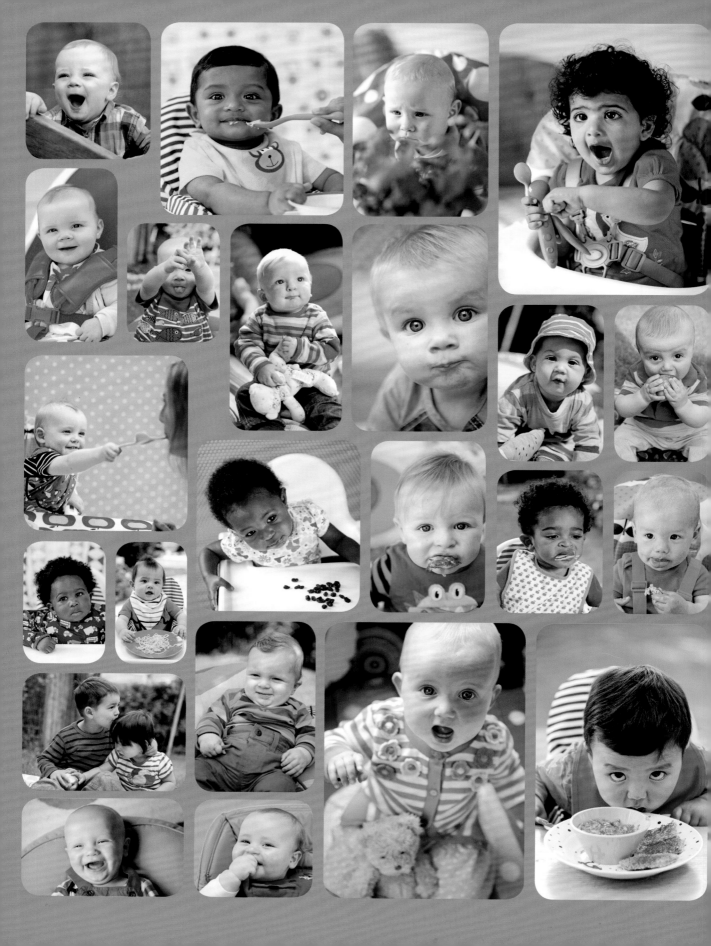

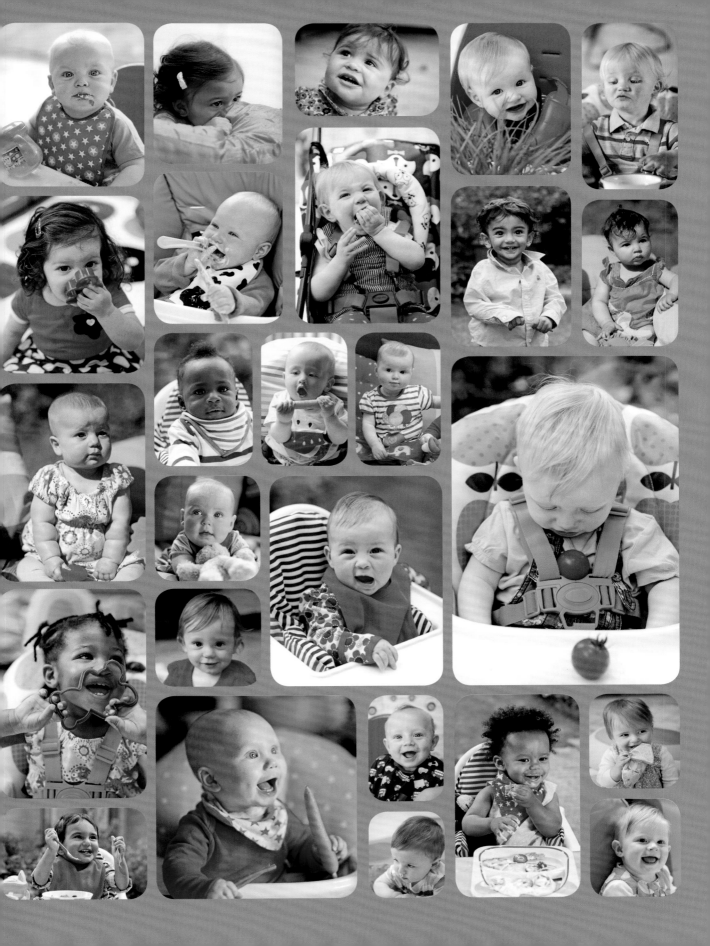

Index

Thank you

A big thank you to all of the Ella's Kitchen employees and friends who contributed recipe ideas for this book and 'road-tested' them with their own families.

A huge thank you to Brother Max, Cosatto, JoJo Maman Bébé, Marimekko, Next, Rice, Skibz and Tomy for their kind supply of colourful clothes and equipment, which helped make our photographs all the more lovely.

A special thank you to all our little helpers – and their parents and carers – for their patience in front of the camera. Here's a list of our little stars and their ages on the days of our photoshoots.

Adriana Bussandri Morais (11 months) • Alex Schembri (3 years) • Amilia Rose Morrison (17 months) • Amy Powell (6 months) • Anima Tavares (11 months) • Austin Van de Peer (12 months) • Benjamin Lee (7 months) • Betsy Swaffer (10 months) • Bruce Burton (7 months) • Carter-Jay Moka (2 years) • Charlie Nichols (11 months) • Creedan-Lee Moka (6 months) • Delphine Wetz (6 months) • Dilan Johal (12 months) • Edie Carter (14 months) • Eloise Mills (6 months) • Eloise-Rose Ludlow-Wade (11 months) • Emilia Kooyman (6 months) • Esha Patel (10 months) • Evelyn Bolton (7 months) • Florence Pallent (7 months) • Freya Phoenix Kelly (10 months) • Harriet King (9 months) • Harrison McDonnell (7 months) • Harry Belmore (10 months) • Holly Crawford (10 months) • Hugo Tang (7 months) • IreOluwa Ade-Onojobi (7 months) • Jack Jensen-Humphreys (17 months) • Jai-Han Marshall (11 months) • Jasmine Layla Bryan (13 months) • Jessica Laycock (9 months) • Joseph Bartlett (6 months) • Joseph Cartlidge (7 months) • Joshua Davis (7 months) • Katharine English (8 months) • Luther Morgan (8 months) • Matilda Friend (8 months) • Matilda Schembri (11 months) • Max McGinty (14 months) • Moshmi Bhagat (16 months) • Oliver Belmore (2 years) • Oscar Brennan (10 months) • Otto White (12 months) • Reuben Nash (7 months) • Rhys MacQueen (13 months) • Ruben Brown (6 months) • Rupert Gillett (18 months) • Sam English (2 years) • Samarth Dhawan (11 months) • Sienna Johal (5 years) • Taliesin Swift (9 months) • Una Gormley (16 months)

And to the mums, dads and grandparents that let us take photos of them, too:

Anna-Louise Lee • Becky Kernutt • Bernadette Ward • Danielle Brown • Donna Clarke • Ellie Wetz • Gemma Moore • Jason Morrison • Karen Kooyman • Leona Melius • Manjinder Johal • Michelle Moka • Moji Ade-Onojobi • Patsy Morse • Samantha Dhanilall

For all the advice in 'Our friends say…', thank you to the following parents and their inspirational little ones:

Angie Turner (Reece + Summer) • Belinda Middleton (Isaac + William) • Bethany Clinton (Sebastian + Jude) • Caitlin Wales (Isla) • Hannah Llywelyn-Davies (Sion + Florence) • Jo Matthews (Samuel + Evie) • Kaela Moore (Cayden) • Katie Green (Lucie) • Katrina Minoletti (Toby) • Kirsten Shepherd (Jessica) • Lottie Ainsworth-Moore (Tabitha) • Megan Sawyers (Rose) • Melanie Almenhali (Mariam, Assia + Ryan) • Natasha Tenpow (Charlie) • Nicole Borbely (Cameron + Oliver) • Nicole McDonnell (Callum + Harrison) • Pamela Newby (Paige) • Photini Konnarides (Danny + Aurelia) • Rhiannon Patel (Fox) • Sophie Harper (Tristan + Alice) • Vicki Cullen (Tilly)

For letting us take photos at their homes, and for all of the other important stuff we needed for our First Foods Book:

Angie Turner, Anita Mangan, Celia Huxtable, Claire Baseley, Emily Quah, Eve and Andy Pallent, Fredderick Karabela, Judy Barratt, Lincoln Jefferson, Manisha Patel, Natasha Field, Rosie Reynolds, Sam Burges, Sarah Ford, Sophie Bristow Symonds, Val Mote and Victoria Cripps

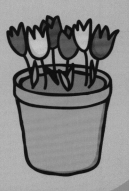

192